Fait

OVERCOMING
RUNAWAY
BLOOD
SUGAR

OVERCOMING RUNAWAY BLOOD SUGAR

DENNIS POLLOCK

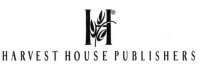

HARVEST HOUSE PUBLISHERS

EUGENE, OREGON

Cover by Koechel Peterson & Associates, Inc., Minneapolis, Minnesota

Back-cover author photo © Larry Watts

Advisory

Readers are advised to consult with their physician or other medical practitioner before implementing the suggestions that follow.

This book is not intended to take the place of sound medical advice or to treat specific maladies. Neither the author nor the publisher assumes any liability for possible adverse consequences as a result of the information contained herein.

OVERCOMING RUNAWAY BLOOD SUGAR

Copyright © 2006 by Dennis Pollock
Published by Harvest House Publishers
Eugene, Oregon 97402

Library of Congress Cataloging-in-Publication Data

Pollock, Dennis, 1953–
Overcoming runaway blood sugar / Dennis Pollock.
    p.   cm.
Includes bibliographical references.
ISBN-13: 978-0-7369-1721-6 (pbk.)
ISBN-10: 0-7369-1721-7
1. Blood sugar—Popular works. 2. Blood sugar monitoring—Popular works. 3. Insulin resistance—Popular works. 4. Diabetes—Prevention—Popular works. 5. Health—Religious aspects—Christianity—Popular works. I. Title.
    QP99.3.B5P65 2006
    612.1'2—dc22   2005018233

Printed in the United States of America

06 07 08 09 10 11 12 13 14 / DP-MS / 10 9 8 7 6 5 4 3 2 1

I am fearfully and wonderfully made;
Your works are wonderful,
I know that full well.

—Psalm 139:14

Contents

Foreword

Dennis Pollock knew his body was telling him something. Feeling weak and shaking like a car running on fumes, he came to realize that despite the fact he had eaten recently, his tank was empty. In this book he shares with you his determination to get to the bottom of his problems with hypoglycemia (low blood sugar) and then do something about it.

Dennis sought to investigate what was happening, to find the malfunction. He learned about the body's ingenious, God-given systems for processing sugars. And in the following chapters he explains what he found out and offers a commonsense approach to changing your behavior so your lifestyle can work in harmony with your body's design.

If you put sugar in the gas tank of the best of our machines, from a Mercedes automobile to the Space Shuttle, it will destroy them. It turns out the human body is no different. This great metabolic masterpiece, this engineering marvel, is being undone by neglect and abuse. We have literally been pouring sugar in our gas tanks. Even though we use glucose as fuel, we have overloaded the tank and overwhelmed the system.

And we continue to do so at a record pace and in record numbers. A 12-ounce cola has approximately nine teaspoons of sugar. Of course, we rarely drink only 12-ounce colas anymore. The size of soft drinks has continued to increase, and it is not unusual to see people walking around carrying 44-ounce behemoths. As a result, statistics show we have more than doubled our soft-drink consumption over the last 25 years. Further, we super-size everything—the serving sizes of tacos, french fries, cheeseburgers, and pizzas have grown correspondingly with the increased appetite and body size of those who consume them. We are in the midst of a carbohydrate crisis.

What is more, the high carbohydrate loading caused by the consumption of simple sugar results in *rebound hypoglycemia*. This low-blood-sugar state following meals manifests itself in fatigue, with decreased energy and decreased productivity. Our lives are, therefore, less than they should be.

More dangerous, however, is the body's long-term response to these high sugar loads. Men, women, and children are subjecting their bodies to glucose loads that were never intended by their Creator. After years of handling increased serum glucose, the pancreas can become unable to produce insulin at levels necessary to handle the work of moving the glucose into the cells. Further, people begin to develop insulin resistance in these situations—as the body becomes less sensitive to the insulin that is produced.

As a result, the disease of diabetes mellitus has reached epidemic levels. The "runaway blood sugar"—uncontrolled serum-glucose levels—seen in persons with diabetes causes severe "end-organ" damage—resulting in, among other things, kidney failure, nerve damage and blood-vessel disease in the extremities, coronary-artery disease, and blindness. Diabetes mellitus is listed as the sixth-leading cause of death. The costs of this disease to the United States taxpayer are staggering. Recent estimates put the tab at approximately 132 billion dollars per year. (Of course, the costs in human terms cannot be calculated.)

There's Something You Can Do About It

As a physician, I have witnessed firsthand, and all too frequently, the ravages of unchecked diabetes. Of course, in many respects it is not unlike other disease states with which we are familiar. Diabetes, heart disease, and cancer often have both genetic and behavioral components to them. We are born with inherited genetics we can currently do precious little about. Our bodies are destined to fail, wear out, fall apart, or succumb to one of the many infirmities that exist in the world.

The good news is, we are able to affect the behavioral component of this condition. Through our actions we are able to extend our life and to be healthier during the years we are given.

What price can you put on your health? On your eyesight? On ten more years of life with your loved ones? Fortunately, by making changes in key areas of your life, you can chart a course toward good health. Dennis Pollock is offering practical advice to help you move toward this healthy living—living more abundantly.

—*Lee A. Brock, M.D.*

The Face of a Giant

It kills more Americans in one year than several dozen World Trade Center attacks. It not only kills—it maims, it cripples, and it blinds. It's diabetes. Along with its precursor, hypoglycemia (both are blood-sugar afflictions), it is making life miserable for millions.

I was well on my way to succumbing to it. In the fall of 2001 my blood-sugar system began to break down. The whole thing was terrifying—it seemed like a giant that was unbeatable.

However, giants may be big and terrifying, but they can be beaten. This book chronicles the insights I gained along the way as I saw the giant fall.

CHAPTER ONE

Christmas Scare

It should have been a pleasant night. It was the Christmas season, and we had just returned from our annual Christmas trip to Grandma's house. We were sitting in our living room, watching a videotape that was one of my sons' Christmas presents.

I wasn't having fun. It was happening again. Less than three hours after we had eaten supper I could feel that cold chill on my arms and those jittery telltale indicators that my blood-sugar levels were falling way too low. I quietly slipped out of the room and went into the bathroom to check my blood sugar with my glucometer—a device I had been totally ignorant of a year earlier but was now all too familiar with.

As I suspected, my blood-sugar level was dangerously low, so low I knew I needed to take action fast. Grabbing a can of Coke, I drank the entire contents in under a minute. Now my blood sugar went the other way. Another test revealed the level had gone from 40 mg/dl to about 170 in a very short time.* (The normal range is 80 to 120.) My body began to tremble violently. I tried to go back into the living room and watch the movie, hoping no one would notice the trembling, but I realized the shaking wasn't going to go away very soon. I slipped into the bedroom, put on a music CD, and got under the covers. As I trembled and shook, I could only think, *What in the world is wrong with me?*

Looking Back

The Christmas scare was not my first encounter with blood-sugar problems. As I look back over my life now, I realize I have had blood-sugar issues going back to the mid-1980s. In the early days I could not have identified them as such; I just knew that when I ate a large pancake breakfast with lots of syrup on Saturday mornings, I felt a little jittery by late morning. It didn't stop me from eating the pancakes, and I just assumed it was "one of those things."

Many times I noticed that when I would go several hours without food I would get that "nervous feeling." My handwriting, already pretty bad, would deteriorate to the point where it was hardly legible. I knew these things were related to food, but I wasn't sure just how it all worked or what, if anything, I could do about it.

---

* Mg/dl = milligrams per deciliter, the standard measuring unit for blood-sugar level. (A deciliter is one-tenth of a liter.)

When I reached the age of 40 things started getting pretty serious. I went through a period where I would feel like I was about to faint if I ate something extremely sugary. Once, at a grocery store I had to run to the car for fear I would pass out on the floor. I sat in the car and waited for my body to return to normal. I began to wonder if I had, or was in the process of getting, diabetes.

I immediately took some steps to try to fix the problem. I cut out nearly all sweets from my diet and began to take jogging more seriously. I soon got better—and after a while went back to my old habits.

During all this time I was very much ignorant of the nature of blood-sugar problems, as well as of why they occurred and what could be done about them. My attempts at reducing sugar in my diet and jogging were certainly steps in the right direction, but they were more intuitive than from a basis of knowledge. Because I didn't know what was going on with my body, it was hard to continue with the changes I had begun.

A Real Danger Signal

It took about eight years for my body to finally get to the point where I became desperate to find some answers. The shakiness that had been a sporadic problem for the previous 20 years or so returned again, and this time with a vengeance. I finally had the breakdown that got my attention and convinced me I had a real problem. I was in church when it happened. Attempting to quietly slip out of the sanctuary just before the service ended, I stumbled and twisted my ankle. In pain I hobbled out of the auditorium and made my way to the wall. I felt that strange sensation that tells you you are losing control of your body. I put my back against the wall and slid down to the floor.

The next thing I knew, several people were hovering over me. I had fainted. The paramedics had been called, and there was nothing to do but wait for them. When they arrived I told them this might be a blood-sugar problem. They immediately asked if I was a diabetic, and I told them I wasn't but I had had low blood sugar at times.

They quickly produced a glucometer and checked me. The device hardly registered! I asked for some food, and I began to eat everything they could find for me. Orange juice, animal cookies from the nursery—it didn't matter.

After a few minutes the paramedics checked my blood sugar again. This time it read 76. This was still pretty low, considering what I had just eaten, but at least was in the safe range. They tried to get me to go to the hospital, but I refused—and after the humiliating experience of being taken out to my car in a wheelchair, I sat in the passenger side, confused and shaken, as my wife drove me home.

Dangerous Plans

I should have gone to a doctor at this point, but I didn't.* Instead I went to the Internet. I did all kinds of searches, using such words as "low blood sugar," "diabetes," "reversing diabetes," and so forth. There had to be something I could do!

One of the first sources of information I found nearly

---

* Here I urge you *not* to follow my example. Good background knowledge is important and motivating, but if you suspect you have blood-sugar problems, it's very important to be under a doctor's care.

did me in. I began to read of a program that was supposed to "reverse diabetes" through exercise and a high-
carbohydrate diet. I wasn't sure I had diabetes, but I knew
I either had it or was on the verge of getting this dreaded
disease. The program's developer was the head of a
diabetes institute that held seminars all over the country
and touted a high-carb, nearly vegetarian diet. He gave
impressive statistics about people he had been able to
help, and he wrote very authoritatively.

Convinced this must be the way to go, I immediately began a radical change of diet. I eliminated almost
all meat and began to limit my foods to mostly carbs,
supplemented by a few vegetables. Beans on bread, bean
soups, bean burgers, rice, spaghetti (no meat added to the
sauce)—these became my "manna." (It was a "carb, carb
here, and a carb, carb there—here a carb, there a carb,
everywhere a carb, carb"...)

My blood-sugar problems immediately multiplied.
By this point I had a glucometer and was testing myself.
I found my blood-sugar level dropping precipitously
at times. I was getting to the point where I was eating
constantly just to keep the bottom from dropping out of
my levels. I began having very strange physical sensations
throughout the day. I wasn't sure just what was going on,
but I knew things were definitely not right.

During this time the fear of diabetes was constantly
with me, a voice that whispered I was heading for a life of
misery and early death. My mother, who had passed away
by then, had suffered from diabetes the last 25 years of
her life. She had had both legs amputated and had experienced all kinds of physical maladies in her later years. I

seemed to be going in the same direction, only getting an earlier start. It was not a pleasant prospect.

Starting to Find Answers

Finally I broke down and went to a doctor. Not being a diabetes specialist, she was not able to give me the answers I needed. She did tell me that at this time, my fasting blood sugar was not at diabetic levels, and she advised me to add some protein to my diet to help stabilize my blood sugar. I began to add some meat to my diet, and sure enough, I had fewer episodes of falling blood sugar. Still, my readings were all over the place, sometimes well above normal, other times well below—even dangerously low.

An Answer to Prayer

Because I am a Christian I had been praying for healing during the health struggles I'm telling you about. Knowing that God could instantly heal me, I figured that would be the best way for Him to answer my prayers. One quick zap—and I could go back to eating as I always had and forget about the whole miserable business. The zap did not come. (I still believe in "zaps," but God is not our bellboy. He heals in His time and in His way.)

Things began to change when I happened to notice a magazine that had come to our office, produced by the doctor whose high-carb solution to diabetic symptoms had about killed me. I noticed in it a number of outrageous claims, such as a report that someone in Texas had found a cure for cancer. Red flags began to go up. This and other claims and promises convinced me that this guy was the medical establishment's equivalent to the *National Enquirer*. I decided it was time to do some more research.

I had a very simple way to test the various theories I encountered. My trusty glucometer could tell me how my body felt about the foods and lifestyles I was imposing upon it. As I did more tests, I began to figure out that my blood sugar would typically peak about an hour after I had finished a meal. That seemed to be the natural time to take a reading, as it would tell me just how acutely my body was reacting to a particular meal.

On one of my ministry trips, I determined to check my blood sugar after nearly every meal. A lunch consisting of a large hamburger (with a large bun) and several handfuls of Fritos led to a reading of 180—much too high. About an hour later the reading was in the normal range, indicating that my pancreas was still putting out insulin, but that my body was slow in dealing with the carbs that turn into sugars.

Another meal I had on that trip was a chef salad with chicken strips. About an hour later I found that my blood-sugar level had hardly risen; it was well within the normal range. As I thought over the difference between my readings after those two meals, I began to feel a sense of hope. Apparently the food that I put into my body had a dramatic effect. Now this is no great revelation to those who study diabetes and hypoglycemia. It is very much common knowledge. But for me it was a wonderful enlightenment. It was empowering to think I could make decisions that affected blood sugar. Some of the mystery was being removed.

Since that time, having taken countless blood-sugar readings and read extensively on the issues of blood-sugar problems and diabetes, I have found some keys that have worked incredibly in my own life. The rest of this book is devoted to sharing those keys with you, which will give you the knowledge you need to literally change your physical destiny.

A View Down the Road

If you are reading this book, it is likely you have some form of blood-sugar problems. These can range from slight jittery feelings when you eat sugary foods and then go too long without eating again, to having a severely elevated blood-sugar level that is destroying your health and will eventually take your life. The remedy should be in keeping with the need.

What are some of the things you can expect to find in the coming chapters of this book? And what are the kinds of changes you will want—or need—to consider to bring your blood-sugar problems under control?

For the Mildest Cases

If your problems are in the "mild" category, you may not want to get as radical as others who are in a more severe situation. People who fit in this category have normal fasting blood-sugar levels (80 to 100) and never see their blood-sugar level rise above 145 or so. Avoiding most desserts, cutting back on potatoes, and limiting your bread to whole-wheat may be sufficient. (The South Beach diet is an excellent guideline to follow.)

Let a glucometer be your guide. Remember, though, that blood-sugar woes are progressive. People do not go from normal to raging diabetics overnight. Those shaky feelings you get when you go too long without eating are a warning sign to you. They would not be happening if your blood-sugar mechanisms were running like a well-oiled machine. Things are starting to break down. The tricky part of this is, the rate of breakdown can be very different for different individuals. Some people's systems can degenerate very slowly, and they can stay in the mild range for decades. Others find themselves on a slippery slope, which could lead rapidly to a disastrous diabetic condition.

The one thing that helps is knowing that when you move toward a low-carb lifestyle you are simply doing what you should have been doing all along. Stuffing your mouth with french fries, downing enormous amounts of Coke, and constantly grazing on doughnuts and jelly rolls is not a natural condition. (Even the high-carb, low-meat guys will admit that much.) So why take a chance and try to live as close to the edge as possible, hoping that diabetes will not strike? Bring those appetites under control and let moderation be your watchword.

Medium Cases

I would include myself in the medium-case category (although my personal diet is more radical than I am here recommending). With medium blood-sugar problems you may or may not have an elevated fasting blood-sugar

level, but your body does not react well to large doses
of sugar or carbs of other kinds. Your pancreas is probably still doing its job, but your body just doesn't process
the insulin it produces very well. And so, without dietary
changes your pancreas will be vastly overworked. Unless
you make changes, you have high chances to become a
diabetic. Although you don't realize it, your body is filled
with insulin nearly all the time, trying vainly to keep
up with the demands you are placing on your worn-out
blood-sugar system. All that insulin isn't doing your heart
any good, either!

If you are in such a position, start consulting with
your doctor if you haven't already. It would be good for
you to get a glucose tolerance test, which will most likely
confirm what you already suspect—you don't tolerate
glucose well. Even small amounts raise your blood-sugar
level, and large amounts send it into the stratosphere.

You will need to do more than merely cut out desserts
and eat smaller portions of the high-carb foods. For the
rest of your life you will need to be consciously and
continually aware of the carb potential of each meal. You
must determine that white-flour products and sugary
foods are a thing of the past. You will need to be careful
even with the "good" carb foods, such as beans, brown
rice, and whole-wheat bread. Sure, you can spoil yourself
once in a while with a small helping of a rice dish, or a
bowl of beans, or half a portion of fruit. But there's no
getting around it—your diet, for the rest of your life, is
going to have to be different from other people's (until
our society gets up to speed in its knowledge of low-carb
eating).

Severe Cases

The severe cases are the full-fledged diabetics, those who require medication or insulin shots to keep their sugar levels somewhere close to normal. First of all, I cannot emphasize enough that you should see a doctor. Diabetes is nothing to play around with—your life is on the line. Find a doctor you are comfortable with—hopefully one who will encourage a lifestyle change along with the medication he or she prescribes. As you make dietary and other changes, you will need to be very careful to stay on top of what these are doing to your blood-sugar levels.

Two Types of Diabetes

Type 1 diabetes (or insulin-dependent diabetes) occurs when the pancreas is unable to produce insulin. It is caused by the destruction of the beta cells in the pancreas by the body's immune system. It usually develops in childhood or adolescence but may appear at any age.

Type 2 diabetes (or non-insulin-dependent diabetes) occurs when the pancreas does not produce enough insulin to meet the body's needs or the insulin is not metabolized effectively. Type 2 diabetes is usually treated through diet and exercise, although some people must also take oral medications or insulin.

You need to make some fairly radical changes in your diet if you are to achieve the kind of stability that will enable you to live without the kinds of diabetic complications that can absolutely ruin your life. Many otherwise great foods, such as potatoes, certain fruits, whole-wheat breads, cereals, and so forth, are going to need to be greatly reduced for the sake of your health.*

Let me add that, for type 2 diabetics on medication, there is still an excellent chance you may be able to get off the medication and control your blood sugar through diet and exercise. Don't do this automatically! Keep a close check on your blood-sugar levels, and keep in close contact with a doctor. But you will never know whether you can be free of your medication if you don't give a low-carb diet a chance. And even if you still need medication, it is almost certain you will be able to go to a lower dosage, which will be a great boon to your health and your chances for longevity.

I have written this book primarily for those who are actual or potential type 2 diabetics, but let me say a word to my type 1 friends: One thing you must not do is simply take your insulin and eat however you will. You must take control of your diet! It is pure deception to think your insulin shots make dietary control unnecessary. The worse your diet, the more insulin you will need—and the more insulin you put into your body, the more you will eventually damage it. There is simply no way you can maintain control of your blood sugar when you are constantly ingesting pancakes, jelly rolls, baked potatoes, biscuits

---

* For type 1 diabetics (whose pancreas is producing no or almost no insulin) I would strongly recommend you purchase, read, and reread *Dr. Bernstein's Diabetes Solution* by Dr. Richard Bernstein. This is a great testimony by a man who should have died years ago of his diabetes, but instead has lived to a ripe old age and has found the keys to good health despite producing virtually no insulin on his own.

and gravy, cakes, pies, and the like.* Your goal is not to eat high-carb meals and then quickly bring your levels down with a shot, but to eat low-carb meals and then supplement your body's insulin deficiency through medication to keep your blood sugar in a healthy range all day long.

The Past, the Present—and a Hopeful Future

The simple truth is, our bodies do not work as well as we reach middle age. As youths we could polish off a meal of pancakes with lots of syrup, have a large glass of orange juice, and then eat a candy bar for "dessert." Our pancreas would squirt out a little insulin, and our cells, bursting with the power of youth, would deal quickly and efficiently with the large doses of sugar and carbs we had ingested. We gave no thought to the fact that 40 years of mistreating our bodies in this way would eventually produce major health issues. We were young, life was good, and all was well with the world.

However, he that would dance the dance must pay the fiddler. After devouring literally thousands of pounds of sugar, white flour, candy bars, ice cream, pies, cakes, and the rest, our bodies gradually lost the efficient metabolism we enjoyed in youth. Now, with our sedentary lifestyles and with carrying more weight than we should, the problem is made worse. We begin to notice "sinking feelings," sugar highs, jittery nerves, and other physical

---

* It is possible to even end up as a "double diabetic." By this I mean that you not only are diabetic in the sense of your pancreas producing little or no insulin, but your body is also becoming highly insulin-resistant, resulting in the need for higher and higher doses of insulin to maintain normal blood-sugar levels. Eventually normal levels can become impossible, even with huge doses of insulin.

manifestations. We are well on the road to major health crises, which can include hypoglycemia, diabetes, heart disease, clogged arteries, and numerous other maladies. The fiddler must be paid.

There is good news, though. The effects of much of the damage you have inflicted upon yourself can be reversed, or at least greatly lessened. *There is hope for you!* Stability is the goal. Soaring highs and plunging lows in blood sugar are the enemy that must be overcome.

You don't have to accept diabetes as inevitable just because one or both of your parents had it. You don't have to live with blood-sugar fluctuations that make your life miserable. There are steps you can take. Diabetes and blood-sugar extremes are not some divine plan sent to you from heaven. As you cooperate with certain basic physical laws, you will be amazed at how your body responds. You can alter your future!

PART ONE

Where We're At

CHAPTER 2

What's Wrong with the American Lifestyle?

In the area of health, America has a lot going for it. We have health and fitness clubs in nearly every city. We have medical technology and understanding such as our forefathers could never have dreamed of. Health and nutrition books pour off our printing presses by the ton. Fitness and health gurus with slim, tan bodies and winsome personalities appear on television to lead us into the promised land of well-being. Many Americans have health insurance that enables them to run to the doctor at the slightest twinge of pain or trace of physical malady and have themselves thoroughly checked out at almost no cost to them. Brain scans, full-body X-rays, blood tests of every kind, and all sorts of other measures are routinely used to diagnose problems at their earliest stages.

Polio and smallpox have been eliminated, the black death is no more, and even cancer is not the death sentence it once was. As a result our average life span is slowly and steadily increasing. It's a great time to be an American. We work shorter hours, enjoy more luxuries, eat a greater variety of foods, and live longer than our grandparents did.

Yet something is wrong. Our increased life span is a bit of an illusion. Because we have been so successful in combating infectious diseases, and because we have such better means of preserving the lives of infants in their fragile states, the numbers don't really tell us what we think they do. Here is a baby that, because of our increased technology and superior knowledge, lives through a crisis that would have taken his life 60 years ago. So instead of dying at three months he lives to the age of 69 before dying of a heart attack.

You can see what a few such cases in every community would do to the national averages. By cutting the mortality rate of infants and doing away with such things as smallpox and polio, we have enabled people to add many decades to their lives and have radically changed the average life span for our nation. But if you ignore these factors, you will find we really haven't improved at all. In fact, we actually have far more people dying of heart attacks and strokes today than in the days of our great-grandfathers. If someone from that generation managed to live through their infancy and avoided infectious diseases, they had an excellent chance of outliving most of us!

It takes just a little research to realize there have been, and still are, what we would call "primitive societies" that are nearly free of heart attacks and diabetes. This is no accident. It follows that, unless they are drinking some pretty special water, there must be something in the lifestyle and diet of these people that has had a radical effect in preventing certain diseases. They may have bad teeth; they may know little about immunization shots or aerobics; but they are doing something very, very right. If we can isolate what it is they are doing (or not doing) that leads to such results, we will gain a treasure of great value.

Something Can Be Done

If you are to stay on course with the lifestyle changes I'm recommending, you must come to see that the typical American lifestyle is both unnatural and unhealthy. This should be self-evident. Considering how many advantages we have over every other society that has ever existed on the planet, we are dying way too early, and we are living much too sickly. Americans' bodies typically begin breaking down in their late 40s or early 50s. This is not to say that you are ready for the grave by then, but it is at this time that the excesses of the standard American lifestyle begin to take their toll.

Things are not getting any better. For several decades the medical establishment has been touting the benefits of a low-fat, high-carb diet. Americans have dutifully moved in this direction. The problem with this kind of diet is that it actually encourages people to consume vast quantities of sugar and white-flour products. After all, if fat is the bad guy, then it must be okay to eat lots of spaghetti, and other pasta, and doughnuts, and bagels, and cinnamon rolls. We eat less meat than before, but we consume far more sugar and white flour than ever in our nation's history.

As a result we are fatter than ever, and diabetes is a raging epidemic, having dramatically increased in the last 30 years. And what was once called *adult-onset diabetes* (type 2 diabetes) is now showing up in teens and even elementary-school-age children. Americans have assumed that as long as our diet is low-fat, everything else is fair game. Stay away from meat, and lap up the sugar. We are killing ourselves with sweets.

The knowledge that America is producing more and more diabetics at earlier and earlier ages has one encouraging component. The good news is this: If the way we are eating and living is promoting blood-sugar problems, it must follow that if we can find a way to change our lifestyle we can vastly improve our blood-sugar situation. Diabetes, hypoglycemia, and other blood-sugar afflictions are not things that providentially fall upon us out of heaven. We can exercise significant control over them. If there are societies that have not suffered from blood-sugar problems, we can hope to find out why, duplicate those factors in our own lives (in an "Americanized" version), and hope to see a major breakthrough in our own health.

Just Who's Weird?

The American lifestyle is both unnatural and unhealthy. Knowing this gives us the courage to forsake it and choose a wiser way of life. We are not being forced to give up some blessing of God and live lives of privation henceforth. We are simply moving toward a way of life that is eminently reasonable. We are not the odd ones (though people will surely make you feel that way!). It is the pizza-gorging, doughnut-eating, cola-drinking, pretzel-snacking, white-bread-stuffing world that's out of step.

We've already touched on the factors in the American way of life that are wreaking such havoc on our health and our delicate blood-sugar mechanisms. Let's take a closer look at the big three.

Problem #1: Sedentary Lifestyle

God created our bodies to be used. In fact, the importance of *use* seems to be a universal principle that applies to everything, not just our bodies. Consider these words of Jesus:

> Whoever has, to him more will be given, and he will have abundance; but whoever does not have, even what he has will be taken away from him (Matthew 13:12).

My paraphrase of this verse would be, "He who uses what he has gets more; he who does not use what he has loses it." Or to put it more simply, "Use it or lose it." This principle is as consistent as gravity and as basic as the law of action and reaction. Arnold Schwarzenegger is a perfect example. How did he get that incredible physique? He didn't get it by watching *Three Stooges* reruns. He got it by using his muscles, and using them, and using them. Our muscles respond to use. The more they are used, the larger and more powerful they become. Weight lifters may start out scrawnier than Barney Fife, but as they keep putting their muscles to use through the constant lifting of weights, they literally build their bodies.

A nursing mother is another example of this principle. When a woman has a baby and begins to nurse, her milk supply is increased or decreased by the demand her baby puts upon her. As the baby develops a greater appetite, the mother's milk is automatically increased. When she stops nursing her milk factory soon shuts down. Lack of use leads to lack of production.

Made for Activity

Our bodies were made for activity. Consider walking. Researchers are beginning to think that this may well be the best exercise of all. For thousands of years people have been walking as their main means of transportation. Horses, donkeys, and such have been useful for longer trips, but walking has been our basic means of getting around from the very beginning.

Physical inactivity is a sure invitation to blood-sugar problems, and eventually full-blown diabetes. There may be a few blessed individuals who have a metabolic consti- tution so strong that they can be sedentary for 80 years and never have a worry about blood sugar, but there are very few. With the advent of such things as cable televi- sion, which lures you to sit lifeless for hours at a time while tempting you with dozens of choices of programs, we are becoming world-class couch potatoes. Add the Internet to this, as well as more and more jobs that involve sitting at a desk or computer, and it is not surprising to see why we are reaping serious health problems despite phenomenal medical progress.

It is imperative to understand that a lifestyle that never makes you sweat or raises your heart rate by any significant degree is both unnatural and unhealthy. You could, of course, give up TV and computers and get a job as a walking mail carrier. On the other hand, it will probably be more practical for you to compensate for a mostly sedentary day by scheduling a period of 30 minutes or more where you *do* raise your heart rate—and even sweat a little (or a lot). In doing this you are not making some major sacrifice. You are simply taking reasonable steps to compensate for the unnatural lifestyle that our twenty-first century technology has thrust upon us. You're not being a martyr here; you're just being sensible. You pay for 23-plus hours of convenience by making your body uncomfortable for a 30- to 45-minute workout.

Why Not?

One of the major justifications many give for not exercising is the old "I am constantly on the move all day long" excuse. There are a couple of problems with this. First of all, it's almost never true. There are some people, like many homemakers, who do move about much of the day. However, if they were to examine their days carefully they would find that they are not in a constant flurry of motion. Many domestic duties, such as ironing, cooking, and so forth, do not call for a lot of motion, but involve activity within a confined space.

Secondly, just moving about is not enough. For exercise to be much good for you, it needs to do several things. It must raise your heart rate; if the day is warm it should make you sweat; and it must be maintained for at least 20 minutes and preferably 30. Forty is ideal. Some people do have jobs that require a lot of movement, but few jobs require that you push your body for 30 minutes or more at a time. Most people in physical jobs are able to do their work in a manner that simply does not tax their body to the point of being a major health benefit. Granted, it is far better to work with at least *some* movement than almost no movement at all, but that is not the exercise that will be of the greatest value. You are going to have to find a way to get your heart rate up and keep it up for about a half an hour a day. This doesn't mean you have to become a world-class athlete or play intense basketball games every day. A brisk walk may be sufficient—but no ambling along!

Problem #2: Diet

Americans have a greater variety of foods, and a greater abundance of food, available than any people in the history of our planet. Meats, potatoes, vegetables, salads, cakes, pies, ice cream, fruits...we have it all.

And we eat it all. Though many Americans eat the obligatory fruits and vegetables to satisfy their conscience, usually it is a small token portion. However, when it comes to the meat, potatoes, pasta, rolls, and desserts, that's when we really and truly go hog wild.

For several decades doctors and "experts" have been telling us the road to good health lies in a high-carb, low-fat diet. We've been told meat is mostly bad, fruits and vegetables are good, and carbs are safe and should be the bulk of our diet. We took this to be a license to eat as much white bread, pasta, cinnamon rolls, and cakes as we like. And we do like!

As a result, Americans are fatter than ever, they are being stricken by diabetes at record levels, and they are experiencing blood-sugar problems in their teens. We are pacifying our dietary consciences by going "low fat" and destroying our blood-sugar systems by stuffing ourselves with carbs, carbs, and more carbs. A diet filled with pasta, white bread, candy, soda pop, cake, pie, and ice cream is utterly unnatural. Never in the history of the earth, until the last century, has man so abused his body to such a large degree.

An Unnatural Development

British surgeon T.L. Cleave studied almost a dozen cultures and determined that coronary heart disease and diabetes were nearly nonexistent in cultures that did not consume refined flour or highly sugared products. In his book *Saccharine Disease: The Master Disease of Our Time,* Cleave showed that only 20 years after a culture adopted sugar and white flour as staples of their diets, these scourges of modern civilization would raise their heads.

We have erred exceedingly in making meat the great monster of our time while giving refined flours and sugar-saturated foods and desserts a free pass. We have sown to the wind and are reaping the whirlwind. It is only as we come to recognize the standard American diet (which could be abbreviated SAD!) as being the unnatural, unhealthy, and disastrous diet that it is, that we can make a choice for a better diet with resolve and determination. When we make a radical dietary lifestyle change, we are not doing anything noble or spectacular; we are simply getting back to a "normal" diet such as our wise and loving Creator intended for us all along.

Problem #3: Weight

Being overweight is not a phenomenon exclusive to our generation; it's just that we have so many more overweight people than ever in the history of mankind! We are eating ourselves into early graves. We have come to accept the middle-age paunch as our rightful due. If we are prosperous and doing well in life, we *should* be a little on the heavy side. Skinny people are either "too nervous" or have not reached "the good life" yet.

However, our bodies function far better, we live longer, our blood pressure stays lower, and our endurance is higher when we carry less weight around. The man or woman who lives with an extra 50 pounds of weight is in an unnatural state. You can get away with it for a few decades, but sooner or later it will catch up to you.

It is vital that you understand this. As long as you justify your extra pounds as your rightful portion of the good life, you will have little inclination to do much about it. But we have it all wrong. We generally don't consider weight a problem until it looks unattractive. At that point we may attempt to do something about it. But the real issue is not how pretty you look—it's how well you manage your body according to the way the Creator has designed it. If your body functioned better covered with gold paint you should paint yourself gold. If the human body achieved its peak performance by eating rusty rivets, then you should have a heaping portion of rivets with your steaks.

Of course, this is not the case. But it is an incontrovertible fact that slim people are healthier and live longer than heavy people as a whole. Somehow, with all of our health clubs, all of our aerobics classes, all of our medical knowledge, Americans have never been so obese, and diabetes has never been so prevalent as now.

Consequences

America's unnatural lifestyle and diet have produced a couple of major consequences that constantly stalk our populace. The first is heart failure. Heart attacks used to be quite rare in America. Until the twentieth century the majority of people who had heart problems were those born with congenital heart defects. Ordinary Americans might die of polio, smallpox, or some other infectious disease, but they weren't at all likely to die of a heart attack.

This is an amazing thought! There's almost no one in America today whose life hasn't been affected by heart disease, either touching them personally or else someone they care about. We have seen so much of it, and bypass and "balloon" surgeries have become so common, we just assume this is how life has to be. It does not! If it can be conclusively demonstrated there are and have been cultures where heart disease was nearly nonexistent, we can be sure that, by the grace of God, we can find our way back to a lifestyle that will enable it to be nonexistent for us. We may not be able to persuade anyone else, but *we* can change.

The lifestyle changes recommended in this book not only have the capacity to do away with your blood-sugar woes; they also can go far in reducing the chances of your dying prematurely of a heart attack or stroke.

The other consequence is, of course, diabetes. For most people, this terrible scourge is nothing more than the natural consequence of unnatural living. For them, the terrible price for living the "American way" is diabetes. True, some have strong-enough constitutions to last them 80 years without full-blown diabetes, but few can escape at least some ill effects from an indulgent lifestyle that Americans have accepted as normal.

Hypoglycemia, blood-sugar jitters, those shaky times— all of these are just warm-ups for the main act, which is diabetes. It cannot be predicted just how long this warm-up period will last, but you are surely headed toward that land of foot sores, insulin injections, blindness, amputations, and premature death. An unnatural way of life is leading to an unnatural way of death.

It's time to get back to eating and living in the manner your loving Creator designed for you. It's not too late. The victory will be well worth the fight.

CHAPTER 3

The Nature of
Your Blood-Sugar System

Your body is an incredible result of engineering by
your Creator. What's behind the DNA of even a single
one of your cells is infinitely beyond the capability of all
man's genius and knowledge. God does good work!

Our bodies were created to be nourished by food. In
His kindness, God created a vast variety of foods and food
combinations that can be of use to us in supplying the
vitamins, proteins, minerals, carbohydrates, and fats that
are necessary for our health and strength. (Aren't you
glad we don't have but one boring choice, such as wheat
bran?)

In addition to the basic foods our Creator has provided
us, we have found ways to modify those foods, combine

them, and otherwise transform them to suit our fancy. And while we have often improved on their taste, we rarely improve on their essential nutrition. Generally, the closer we keep foods to their natural state, the better they are for us.

When food enters our stomach, all kinds of incredible things begin happening within us. Gastrointestinal fluids are called up to break the food down into a pasty liquid from which our intestines can extract needed nutrients. Sugars are quickly absorbed into our bloodstream to provide energy. Vitamins and minerals are snatched up in tiny, seemingly insignificant quantities, and yet they play a powerful role in maintaining health. And all this is going on while we sit back and relax, enjoying the luxurious feeling of being full!

Neglect and Abuse

Our bodies usually function so well in our youth that we give no thought at all to how they work. Everything purrs along beautifully on "automatic pilot." We can eat whatever we want, whenever we want, neglect exercise, and generally abuse our bodies, with no apparent consequences. A couple of bowls of sugary Trix cereal for breakfast, a hot dog, fries, and milkshake for lunch; a large pizza washed down with a super-sized Coke for supper; and no protests from within. And don't forget the pre-bedtime snack of a huge bowl of rocky-road ice cream. We're young, we're healthy, we're—invincible! And we're even slim!

Advance the clock 30 years. Decades of abusing our body have begun to take their toll. We're 40 pounds overweight. We've been growing uneasy over those strange pains in our chest, which are telling us of arteries partly clogged. We find ourselves getting shaky when we eat sugary foods and then go a few hours without more food. We don't have the energy we once had. Unless we make some radical changes we face the certain prospect of getting to heaven much sooner than we had once thought. (Which is not a bad deal, but reaching heaven quickly as a result of our own poor choices is not the best way to get there!)

Understanding the way your body works is half the battle. Most of us have enough of the rebel in us to refuse to be much moved by someone preaching to us to change our behavior without giving some good reasons for the change. For me to stand on a soapbox and scream at all passersby, "Give up the sugar, quit eating white bread, lay off the doughnuts!" is probably not going to make me any friends—and may well increase doughnut sales in the area. This is why people who refuse to read or think much about diet and nutrition are always going to be the toughest cases. They may try to change, but their heart will not be in it. They make great yo-yo dieters and fad followers. They lack the motivation that comes from understanding.

The fact that you are reading this book puts you in another category. You are to be congratulated. With that in mind let us consider the role of the major player in the blood-sugar system: insulin.

Insulin and the Processing of Sugars

The average American knows little about insulin, except that it is what diabetics have to take sometimes. Insulin is vitally important to our health in ways that researchers are just finding out. Your body must have energy. Without energy you become a slug and soon die. Energy is produced by the proper absorption of glucose (blood sugar) by the millions of cells in your body. And how do we get this glucose? We get it from carbohydrates, primarily.

This might lead you to say, "If this is true, the more carbohydrates I eat, the more energy I'll have." It sounds plausible, but nothing could be further from the truth. Keep in mind that people have been eating "natural" foods for nearly 6000 years of recorded history. Candy bars, white-flour products, milkshakes, and the like were unknown until five or six generations ago. Until then people lived on mostly meat, vegetables, and whole-grain products. The common drink has always been water, with beer or wine for special occasions. Milk was a luxury, and soda was nonexistent. In most of these societies heart disease either didn't exist or was extremely rare. In many of them diabetes was nowhere to be found!

As we noted in chapter 2, the fact that there were and still are societies that have almost no cases of diabetes is vitally significant. It tells us blood-sugar problems are not merely the lot of those who are genetically predisposed. It is irrational to think that entire cultures—consisting of millions of people—just happened to have none with faulty genetic wiring. Lifestyle as well as genetics must play a major role in this.

And so it does. Your body does indeed require carbohydrates with which to make glucose necessary for energy. But your system is built so well that it doesn't need enormous amounts. Almost every food has a little carbohydrate in it. Vegetables, cheeses, nuts, berries, and all kind of natural foods contain more than enough carbohydrates for your well-being. But the advantage that these foods provide is, they release their carbs into your bloodstream at a slow and steady rate. While a bowl of Trix dumps its many carbs into your system almost immediately, putting a tremendous strain on your pancreas, a salad puts fewer carbs in your blood and takes its time in doing it.

Whether fast or slow, it is your pancreas's job to oversee the regulation of sugar in your bloodstream. As your food is broken down for the body's use, the pancreas "senses" the level of carbohydrates that is being converted to sugar in your bloodstream. Our all-wise Creator created this little gem of an organ to supervise and oversee the blood-sugar process. As it recognizes the level of carbohydrates and sugar it has to deal with, it secretes the amazing and powerful hormone we call insulin.

Insulin is the policeman that tells the blood-sugar levels, "Thus far and no more." It has a way of limiting the levels by enabling glucose to be received by the body's cells at a higher rate. It works with tiny receptor cells which "drink in" the glucose and put it to use in their particular cell. A meal rich in carbohydrates, such as a large pancake breakfast dripping with sweet maple syrup, is going to result in a whole lot more insulin being produced than, say, a meal of eggs and bacon.

Taxing the Pancreas

Your pancreas was created for yeoman's service. It was made to serve you for 70 to 90 years without a hitch. And for many people it does just that. This was especially true in previous generations when it wasn't taxed the way it is today.

One candy bar or one ice-cream cone is not going to do your pancreas in. It was made extremely sturdy and can take a lot of abuse for a good while. Most people can go years, even several decades, before they begin to notice a problem.

It generally happens like this. As we age, our bodies become less efficient. Our metabolism slows down. It becomes easier to gain weight than to lose it. Our cells' insulin receptors don't work as well as they should. Our increased levels of body fat and decreased muscle tone make for worse and worse insulin processing. It takes far more insulin to deal with the carbs we ingest. Our pancreas gamely does its best to keep up. In our youth a tiny squirt of insulin was more than enough to take care of that doughnut-and-soda breakfast, but now it takes three or four times that amount. Our bodies are filled with insulin almost constantly during our waking hours.

Two Key Terms

There are two medical terms that relate to the situation we're discussing. One is *hyperinsulism*, which means just what you would think. It is a state in which your body is being forced to endure the presence of far too much insulin, which is doing its best to deal with the high-sugar, high-refined-flour diet to which you are subjecting it.

The other term is *insulin resistance*. This simply means your body is becoming less efficient at processing insulin. Your pancreas is still working fine; it just takes far more insulin to keep your blood sugar in line than it should. Depending upon the state of your body, you might stay in this insulin-resistant stage for many years without developing full-blown diabetes, or you might move quickly into the world of the diabetic.

One of the warning signs of *insulin resistance* and *hyperinsulism* (see sidebar) is that jittery, shaky feeling you get when you go very long without eating. What is happening is that when you eat a meal high in carbohydrates, your pancreas, faithful to the end, is trying to oblige by dumping enormous amounts of insulin into your bloodstream. Because you are so inefficient at handling blood sugars, it just keeps pouring out the insulin. Finally, after a couple of hours this enormous amount of insulin has done its job. The blood sugars are safely transported to the body's cells, and things are okay. But not for long. The problem is, you still have a large amount of leftover insulin in your bloodstream. But there are no more carbs being put in for this insulin to "feed on." Therefore it begins to drive your blood sugars abnormally low.

At that point you start feeling shaky and nervous. Your handwriting deteriorates. You feel the need to eat something right away. Typically you reach for a candy bar or something sweet, which makes you feel better temporarily but merely starts the process all over again.

Long-Term Results

As this vicious cycle goes on for years, your pancreas is working many times harder than it was ever supposed to. It can take it for a while. And in some cases it never goes beyond this stage. But frequently the pancreas is "blown out" from overwork. It was working at rates never intended by its Creator. The insulin stops coming or slows down to a trickle. At that point you have a serious problem. You have just entered the world of the diabetic, a world filled with those many ugly complications such as blindness, limb amputations, wounds that never heal, and premature death.

Today the incidence of diabetes is increasing in record numbers. People get it earlier than they ever did, more people get it than ever before, and the blood-sugar problems of hypoglycemia and the like are epidemic. (Because I travel frequently, I often get a chance to talk to people about these things because they are curious about my "strange diet." From my observations, it appears that people of 45 or older are having blood-sugar issues of one kind or another as often as not.)

Because of the three issues we discussed in chapter 2—diet, fitness, and weight—our marvelous blood-sugar system, designed for seven to ten decades of effective use, breaks down after only four or five. We are faced with a terrible struggle in our remaining years as we try to limp along with the help of pills or insulin. As we've seen, the lifestyle we're living, seemingly normal to us, is actually a radical departure from the healthy, active way of life our wise Creator intended for.

There's still plenty of good news, nevertheless. We'll start looking at it in the next chapter.

CHAPTER 4

Good News, Bad News, and Good News

If you have come to the painful realization you do indeed have some fairly serious blood-sugar problems, I have some news for you. Actually, I have good news, bad news, and (more) good news. Let's check it out.

The First Good News

Things are not as bad as they seem. When I first began to suspect I might have diabetes—or be moving in that direction—it was a painful and fearful time for me. My wife was intimidated as well. She didn't even want me to use the word *diabetes*. It wasn't quite as bad a word as *cancer*, but it didn't seem too far from it.

Did I or didn't I? Was I or wasn't I? Refusing to get a full battery of tests (I had no health insurance at the time) left me wondering all the time. I only knew I was going to trust God for my healing and do as much reading as I could to try to find some answers about what was happening to me.

Also good news is that there are steps you can take. We know far more about diabetes and related blood-sugar problems than we ever have before. Much research has been done, and more research is going on right now. Two generations ago a diagnosis of diabetes was pretty much a death sentence. One generation ago it could be somewhat controlled and your lifespan extended, but you were likely to face a myriad of physical problems as you limped your way through life. Instruments to measure blood sugar were reserved only for hospitals and a few very wealthy people—the average American had no way of checking his or her own blood sugar.

Today you can pick up a glucometer and a hundred testing strips for about $60. Using the knowledge available, you can make significant changes in your lifestyle. Not only can you prevent the onset or ravages of diabetes, but you can end up improving your overall health to the point where you may live longer than you ever would have had you not had any blood-sugar problems! In short, by the grace of God, you have an excellent chance of controlling your situation and living the "happily ever after" life to which we all aspire.

Now for the Bad News

Alas, there is some bad news. There are some sacrifices

you will have to make. You cannot continue with the lifestyle you have led from your early years till now. Sacrifices are not fun. (That's why we call them *sacrifices!*) They require a measure of willpower and that other key concept—self-control. For the rest of your days you will have to give more thought to your diet than you ever did before. You will need to find creative ways to exercise and stimulate your metabolism. And you will probably need to lose some weight and learn to keep those pounds off.

A Whole Way of Life

Not only will you need to make some pretty radical changes in your lifestyle, you will need to find a way to make these changes a permanent fixture. We are not talking about some fad diet or crash course that will patch things up so you can go back to the way things used to be. You need to mentally calculate how many years you would like to hang around here on the earth...and then figure the changes you make will last exactly that long.

One of the reasons that diets are such poor instruments of weight loss is that most people who start on them have no plan to make them a lifetime habit. So the diet is entered into enthusiastically. It may even help you to lose a few or a lot of pounds, but the day of reckoning soon comes. It dawns on you that you are absolutely sick of your bananas or your Jenny Craig meals or whatever, and you go back to regular food. You tell yourself you will watch it this time and be careful not to overeat—and at first you are pretty careful, but before long you are back to your old habits. And the weight returns, with a few bonus pounds thrown in. The only diet that really has a chance of succeeding is one you are content to live with for the next 30 to 40 years. And of course the same is true with exercise programs.

Exercise and Garage Sales

I have to confess I am a garage-sale junkie. One of my favorite activities on my days off is to go around to garage sales and look for great deals. (One of my big thrills is to find a $25 item that I know that I can sell on E-Bay for more than $100.) As I search for treasures I am always amazed at just how many exercise machines are for sale. I think exercise machines must be the most common large item you see at garage sales.

The reason is simple: People start exercise programs with the best of intentions, but have never settled it in their minds that the program they are beginning is to be their rule of life for the rest of their days. They begin their exercising with the vague notion of improving their muscle tone or lowering their blood pressure or some other worthy goal...but have no real intentions of doing this or any other exercise for the rest of their lives. As a result, after a few missed days they decide it is too hard to get back into the rhythm of exercise, and they let the machine sit idle. After months of inactivity they realize the unused rowing machine or treadmill or exercise bike is sitting there condemning them—and they sell it at their next garage sale, often for a tenth of the original price!

Two Crucial Decisions

The best hope you have for making a change that will last is to go into that change having first decided it will be for all your life; and secondly, making sure the change is not so radical that it will be impossible to maintain.

You will need to say goodbye forever to the old lifestyle you enjoyed for so many years. It will be a sad farewell. You may often recall those carefree days when you never thought about diet, never worried about exercise, and were in blissful ignorance of the blood-sugar issues we discuss in this book. It was so much easier then. You will long for your former youth, ignorance, and excesses that got you into this trouble you are now in.

You can't go back again, though. You can no longer take your body for granted. What was once on "automatic" is now on "manual." Your situation is one that will call for discipline, self-control, and denial of impulses not in harmony with the Creator's design.

The Good News (Again)

While there are indeed some sacrifices to be made to restore your blood-sugar to normality, they are not something that will make you a freak—or consume so much of your time that you can do nothing but spend your days fretting and worrying over every morsel you eat, constantly doing exercises by the hour, and obsessed with every tiny blood-sugar fluctuation. You do not need to drop out of circulation, nor are you being condemned to eating foods you can't stand or never tasting anything sweet again. Far from it.

Yes, there are adjustments to be made. But considering the benefits you will gain, you should be excited. By taking your health seriously at this stage you have excellent chances of

- losing excess weight and looking and feeling better
- reducing your blood pressure and chances of strokes
- reducing your total cholesterol and triglycerides and chances of heart problems
- avoiding all the complications so often associated with diabetes
- living substantially longer than you would have otherwise

By going to a more natural and self-controlled style of living, you may well enjoy decades of freedom from blood-sugar problems. You can say goodbye to those nasty fluctuations and jittery feelings that come from hypoglycemic episodes. You have a great opportunity to enjoy many years of time with your family, watching your children advance in life, taking your grandchildren to movies (if you can find any decent ones to take them to), and being involved in meaningful activities with your church and your friends. Life can be great, and all the more so when you are not distracted by physical illnesses that make you feel like you are tottering on the brink of an abyss.

Your body is a gift from God. Surely our bodies and our health should be treated as the precious gifts they are! By making some wise choices now, you can purchase for yourself a quality of life that is priceless.

CHAPTER 5

Motivational Issues: Why Change?

When it comes to making behavior changes, motivation isn't merely important; it is everything! In most cases we know what we should do. Often we even know how to do it. We simply don't want to do it strongly enough to overcome some conflicting desire. Thus our lives are filled with good intentions, frequent attempts at change, and frequent failures.

When we do see someone who has made a drastic change in his lifestyle or eating patterns we marvel and wonder, *How'd he do that?* Yet it seems so often to be something for the other guy, not something we could ever do.

A key for victory in this area of runaway blood-sugar

levels is the one I've touched on previously: a change in the way we live. Make no mistake about it. If you keep doing what you always have, you will keep seeing the same things you have always seen. Actually, you will see worse things because you are most likely on a downward spiral. Once your blood-sugar system begins to unravel, it is rare for it to remain static. You will either find a way to bring things under control—or you will experience worse and worse metabolic degeneration.

I once had a meal with a diabetic who was having severe difficulties with his blood-sugar levels. He was on insulin, yet even with powerful doses of this hormone, his blood sugar was still out of control. During the meal we had together, he ate a large slice of white bread and a large dessert (both definite no-no's for people with blood-sugar problems). This man, who was only middle-aged, was passing a sentence of misery upon his remaining years for his lack of self-control. Some way, somehow, you must find the motivation to change your lifestyle. Don't worry. You can find it if you look in the right place.

Changes and Motivation

One of the great mysteries of life is why some people seem to be so much more motivated than others. Just as people are born with varying degrees of talent and beauty, so we find individuals are radically different in motivation. It doesn't take long for this to appear. Go to any first-grade class and you will find certain children who work more diligently and are far more conscientious in their efforts than others. One kid races through an assignment, finishing quickly but producing a paper riddled with errors—while his friend sitting behind him, who is no smarter, puts ten times the effort into it and turns in an outstanding assignment. These children were not trained to be the way they are; no one can explain why the spark of motivation burns brightly in one while hardly appearing in another. Take a look at the life of a biblical writer, the apostle Paul. Here we begin to uncover an answer. He had an overriding goal. In the area of self-discipline he summed up his philosophy in these words:

> I discipline my body and bring it into subjection, lest, when I have preached to others, I myself should become disqualified (1 Corinthians 9:27).

Implied in this declaration is the fact that our bodies need to be controlled; they cannot be given free rein to enjoy whatever they may wish. This should be pretty much self-evident. If you truly gave your body everything it demanded, you would never do any kind of exercise. (What fun is that?) You would eat all kinds of sugary foods and hardly eat any vegetables. (Who would choose brussels sprouts over strawberry shortcake topped with whipped cream?) You would choose white-flour products over whole-wheat. You would eat until you were stuffed. You would grow huge, and your body would begin to experience breakdowns of various kinds. Sounds kind of familiar, doesn't it?

If motivation were something we could buy at Wal-Mart, we'd all have it. But if you are experiencing blood-sugar difficulties, you are going to need some motivation from somewhere. Whatever genes you may have inherited, you are going to have to make some fairly major changes.

It's crystal-clear there's a need for motivation; now let's talk about how you actually get it. In the following pages we'll look at four keys for motivation-building: 1) understanding and knowledge, 2) accountability, 3) joy, and 4) success. The thrilling thing about all this is that there are things *you* can do to increase your level of motivation. Whether you have the "motivation gene" or not, you can succeed!

Key #1: Understanding and Knowledge

Knowledge is a powerful motivator. Nearly every voluntary action we take is based upon a collection of facts and insights. Typically, the more knowledge we possess and the more often we think upon that knowledge, the more likely we will be to act in accordance with it. We were created to respond to the inputs that constantly wash over our minds. What the mind continually absorbs, the will begins to enforce. (This proves true for falsehoods as well as truths.)

People who constantly dwell on a single concept, be it a sport, or making money, or sex, or whatever, are going to need little outward motivation to thoroughly give themselves to it. You can bet Tiger Woods doesn't stop thinking about golf when he drives away from the golf course. Bill Gates doesn't stop thinking computers when he gets home from his office. And Billy Graham didn't stop thinking about people's eternal value to God when he stepped down from the platform at a stadium event.

The simple truth is this: People who never read books about health, never watch TV programs about health, and give almost no thought to health and nutrition issues are going to have a very difficult time making lifestyle changes for the betterment of their health. Without allowing your mind to be continually exposed to the truths that can set you free from your blood-sugar miseries, you will never make it. It will not be enough to quickly read this book, make a few changes, and expect to live happily ever after. You are going to have to make these truths part of you. You are going to have to read and think and learn and think and read and think some more. There are a number of good books that can encourage you along the same lines as this one, but you will have to know what to look for, and you will have to make the time to get them and read them.

Of course I could simply tell you, "Do this and don't do that! Eat this and don't eat that!" Perhaps some of you might even do it for a while. But you will never be able to sustain a lifestyle change merely because someone has preached at you. You must learn for yourself the principles that will give you the victory.

I could give all the principles necessary to cure obesity in a very short article. One page would do it. I could tell overweight people to lay off all sugars and refined breads, and never take second helpings or snack between meals. A few other basic suggestions and commandments and they would have what they would need to lose 20, 40, or 200 pounds. But no diet book would be so presumptuous.

Instead nutrition experts go to great lengths to explain not only what you should do, but why you should do it and how you should do it. They baste your mind with their philosophy of nutrition in the hopes of motivating you to make permanent changes.

So it is with this book. I want to encourage you to read this book slowly and allow it to seep into your consciousness. Don't read it just to find out the basics and get on with things. Savor its truths and allow them to penetrate your heart with the need to truly, completely, and permanently change your physical lifestyle. And once you have read it, read some other books like those I will be recommending, and then reread this one. Too much effort? Not considering the stakes that are involved.

Key #2: Accountability

"How are you doing?" is a question we often ask people we meet, but we usually don't expect much of an answer. When it comes to dealing with blood-sugar problems, you absolutely must find a way to know how you are doing. Extreme blood sugars are exceedingly dangerous, and you cannot afford to risk your life and health by assuming you are doing okay.

In addition to being under a doctor's care, today, with the mighty little glucometer you can measure yourself frequently to assess your physical condition. You absolutely must buy one of these. It is one of the best investments you'll ever make in your life. Your glucometer readings are like the report cards you used to get when you were in school. They tell you how well your program is working.

The first time I used a glucometer I was plenty nervous. I

had been having some severe hypoglycemic reactions and thought there was a very real chance I could be a diabetic. I had read enough to know that normal blood-sugar levels range from readings of 80 (usually in the morning before breakfast) to 120 (about an hour after a meal). What would my blood sugar be? I had fearful visions of seeing it read 300 or 400. I took my first reading—and it was in the 120s, to my tremendous relief. It was almost two hours after I had eaten lunch, however, and so this really wasn't the best time to take a reading.

Making a Difference

In the days and months to come I began taking my blood-sugar readings religiously, almost fanatically. I found that what I ate had a great deal to do with what the little glucometer would tell me. As I realized this, I began to experience a wonderful sense of relief. There were things I could do that would make a tremendous difference! I read more about diabetes and the body's blood-sugar functions, and things started becoming clear to me. I realized what tremendous abuse I had been doing to my body for decades.

Not only did my blood-sugar readings after meals go down as I started my new lifestyle change, even my *fasting* blood-sugar levels started going down. The fasting blood-sugar level is simply the number you get when you test yourself in the morning before you have your first bite of food. It is a kind of cumulative measure of how you and your body have been doing, sugar-wise. If you have been constantly feeding your body loads and loads of sugars and starches, forcing your sugar level unnaturally high throughout the day, your fasting blood-sugar level will rise and rise—and will serve as a "tattletale" that you are not doing very well in the blood-sugar department. As you reverse the process and eat carefully and follow a vigorous exercise program, your fasting blood-sugar level will steadily become lower, patting you on the back for being a good boy or girl.

Levels of Alert

Anyone whose fasting blood-sugar level is over 120 has a real problem and needs to see a doctor. Those whose blood sugar is between 110 to 120 are marginal and should take steps quickly to change their lifestyle. But even people with a fasting blood sugar in the healthy 80 to 100 range may overreact to sugars and need to monitor themselves, especially in terms of how fast and far their blood sugar may rise when they eat a meal high in carbohydrates.

The great thing about your glucometer is that it gives you immediate feedback. You don't have to wonder how you're doing—you can see it with your eyes. And the feedback you receive is a wonderful motivator to increase your efforts. As I took my blood-sugar levels in those early days, it was fascinating to me to see how various meals affected me differently. A low reading an hour after a meal was exhilarating! A high reading was somewhat depressing, but it awakened in me the need to know why it was high as well as the desire to do better. Every meal became an experiment, and my blood-sugar levels improved tremendously as I learned how to eat in such a way as not to tax my pancreas, the organ I had so horribly mistreated for most of my years.

It's Simpler Than It Seems

If the idea of constantly taking your blood-sugar levels sounds kind of gloomy, let me give you some great news. First of all, it is not nearly as bad as it sounds. You don't have to prick your finger by stabbing it yourself. You have a pen-like device that will do it at just the right depth, and you will hardly feel it. The process takes about a minute (as few as five seconds with some meters), and you receive invaluable information. Your glucometer is truly your friend.

Here's some other great news. For those who are not true diabetics but have those hypoglycemic episodes that signal the potential for diabetes, you don't have to keep up a constant regimen of taking your blood sugar many times each day. In my discovery days, I would take my blood sugar three or four times a day. By now I know what works and what does not work for me. I know what I can eat and what I cannot stand too much of. I have worked out an exercise program I can live with. Because of this, I usually don't take my readings more than two or three times a month. Usually at the first of the month I take my fasting blood sugar to get my "report card." A reading in the 80s or low 90s is an "A" for me, and I often don't worry about it until the next month. I may take it again if I go out and eat a meal higher in carbs than usual and want to see just how it affected me. (Of course, a full-fledged diabetic needs to check their blood-sugar levels far more often, as prescribed by their doctor.)

Your glucometer is your accountability partner. There is no way you're going to be able to "snow" him or lie to him. Nor will he lie to you (as long as you do the test properly). Good reports from him are your body's way of saying, "You're on the right track. Keep it up." Bad reports are its way of telling you, "You need to make some more changes." In either case these reports are an absolute necessity for those who want to see victory.

Key #3: Joy

Joy may seem like a strange concept to relate to motivation. In fact, joy is most important. Nothing kills motivation any more effectively than lack of joy. Evidence of this is seen in people who are severely depressed. Their most common attribute is a lack of desire to do anything. People who are greatly depressed usually want to spend most of their time in bed.

While I cannot go into this subject at great lengths here, let me suggest that you who are suffering from depression are going to need to address this issue before you can experience total victory.*

And one other thing. Get involved in some kind of helping, serving, or volunteering, whether feeding the poor, teaching children in Sunday school, or whatever you can find to do. We were made to give out as well as take in. If you dwell only on your problems, you will

---

* Speaking as a Christian, one thing I urge you to do is to draw near to God. Your circumstances may be lousy and there may be very little you can do about them. What you *can* do, though, is come near to Him. He is the Source of joy.

only make matters worse. This may not turn you into a bubbly Rebecca of Sunnybrook Farm, but it can make a significant difference in your "joy level" and mean the difference between success and failure.

Key #4: Success

One of my college professors emphasized an old saying, one I have never forgotten: "Nothing succeeds like success." It sounded kind of silly, but the more I have thought about it, the more convinced I have become that he was right. Little successes are tremendous boosters of our confidence and desire. Establish a few small successes early on, and the larger successes are almost sure to come.

One day, as my wife and I were making the long trip home after visiting relatives, I suggested to her that we both needed to lose weight. She had certainly tried before, but her attempts had always been failures. Her frequently given reason for her failures was that "food tastes sooo good!" In fact, she was so intimidated by her weight at this point that she refused to ever weigh herself. When she would go the doctor, she would not look at the scale and would tell the nurse she didn't want to know her weight!

As we drove that day, we began to brainstorm about what we could do to lose weight. We talked about some of the more "pain-free" things, such as switching from regular sodas to diet sodas, switching from regular salad dressing to low-fat dressing, and so forth. We made a few rules to follow, such as no eating between meals and no second helpings at the table. We would take what seemed a reasonable amount and close up shop after our plate was cleaned.

And we began our new "lifestyle change." This time was different. For one thing I was on board, and it is a well-established fact that behavior change is made much easier when it is done in harness with other people. Secondly, we had purchased a scale, which gave instant feedback. Most importantly, we committed our efforts to God.

The weight began to come off. This was no crash diet. Our basic philosophy was that this "diet" had to be a way of eating we could live with for a lifetime. Had we tried to lose the weight too fast or sacrificed too much, we could never have kept up the pace. We would have been like marathoners who started out in a sprint and exhausted ourselves in the first leg of the race.

When my wife had lost ten pounds or so she was thrilled. She could see tangible results staring at her in the face of that scale. The taste of success was intoxicating. One of the statements she made was, "I didn't think I could do it." Now she was beginning to realize she could indeed "do it." I really believe that by that point the victory was already hers. Losing the additional weight was just a matter of time, faith, and following the rules we had established.

Success has a way of doing amazing things to people. While too much success can lead to pride (it doesn't have to, but often does), too much failure can lead people to simply stop trying.

You are going to need some success to keep you on course. By following the principles of this book and keeping a close eye on your blood-sugar levels, you have excellent chances of seeing a whole lot of success. Rejoice in it. Recognize that your condition does not have to deteriorate; it can improve dramatically. As you see your blood-sugar levels getting back to normal, let it spur you to a lifetime of healthy eating, exercise, weight control, and praise to your God!

PART TWO

What to Do

CHAPTER 6

The Battle Plan

⌒

While a battle plan will need to be personalized somewhat for your particular situation, most of this chapter
will apply to everyone. Remember, this is indeed a battle
you are going to engage in. Your health over the next few
decades is riding on the outcome.

We've already mentioned the three primary fronts on
which the main battles will be fought: diet, exercise, and
weight. Win any one of these battles and you will have
done yourself a lifetime favor. Win two of them and it
will be far better. But if, by the grace of God, you can win
on all three fronts, you will be blessed indeed. For most
people (other than type 1 diabetics) a victory on all three
fronts will lead to a radical improvement in blood-sugar

control, and for many it will bring an end to blood-sugar problems altogether.

Many of you are truly fighting for your lives. You are the best candidates to see total victory because you have more on the line. But you must determine that a partial victory is unacceptable. You must push to win on *all* fronts. Throughout history, the most effective military generals have almost always been totally given to the cause. This must be your attitude as well. If you enter the battle with the idea of cheating a little here and there, and then maybe after you achieve a modest goal, easing up a bit from there, you might as well stop right now. Those who don't throw themselves wholeheartedly into the fight will always end up casualties. This will be just one more failed attempt at a lifestyle change, and it will make any future attempts all the more difficult.

The First Front: Diet

Of the three major fronts in this war for your health and blood-sugar stability, this is no doubt the most important. You must—absolutely must—get control of your eating habits. The old you, with your indiscriminate eating habits, with the snacks and sugar, must "die." The new you will eat to live—and no longer live to eat. For all those with blood-sugar problems, this means a low-carbohydrate diet.

One of the key concepts, especially in the early stages of your new lifestyle, is planning. Destructive behavior is usually the result of poor planning or no planning at all. People overspend because they go to stores and just browse. Without a definite objective they are easily overcome by every little "goodie" that their eye lights upon. It is also true in the area of nutrition. Most Americans simply eat whatever they like. They shop for whatever seems appealing, with little thought of a definite nutritional goal. A cake is on sale at the deli, so they buy it. You can't pass up that kind of a bargain, can you?

Thinking Ahead

Yes, you can, and you must think ahead. Not only must you become a disciplined eater, but you must become a disciplined shopper as well. You must think out your meals ahead of time and be able to come up with a great variety of meals that will not overtax your blood-sugar system.

The same is true of snacks. It is natural for us to get hungry between meals, and there is nothing wrong with having an in-between-meal snack at times, as long as it is not loaded with sugar or calories. But if you wait until hunger pains hit and then start to try to figure out what type of snack to have, you are in trouble. Plan ahead! Be prepared mentally and food-wise for snacks. This is also true of regular meals. You must think these things through beforehand. If you wait until the pressure is on to come up with something, you are likely to revert to an old familiar favorite, but one that is not a friend to your body.

It will be important to determine the level to which you are going to reduce your eating of carbohydrates. Every person with blood-sugar problems needs to achieve a significant reduction of carbs, but not everyone needs the same level of reduction. A person with full-blown diabetes, whose pancreas is putting out very little or no insulin, probably needs the greatest reduction. The individual whose pancreas is still putting out enough insulin to keep their fasting blood sugar at a decent level (80 to 105 in the morning before the first meal) can get by with a lesser reduction.

Your glucometer will tell you how serious your state is, and your doctor will help guide you. It is important you set reasonable and attainable goals for yourself. If you have only the slightest symptoms of blood-sugar problems and attempt to maintain a severe diet, you will have an almost impossible time of maintaining it. It would be far better for you to establish a more moderate dietary change and stick with it than go whole hog and fall by the wayside.

Go in braced for challenges. They may come from friends and family who will, with the best of intentions, suggest you are being a fanatic and need to lighten up. There will be times when you will be at people's homes and they will serve something you know you must not eat. In such cases, you can either 1) take such a minuscule portion that it won't make any difference, or 2) explain that you do not eat those things anymore and tell them why.

Encouragement

As a traveling evangelist and Bible teacher, I frequently eat meals at the homes of people I don't know well. I often end up telling them the story of my blood-sugar problems and the answer God has given me. About half the time I find that at least one of my hosts has struggled with blood-sugar problems also and is very interested in finding out more about my diet. I end up making "converts" along the way. It turns out to be a great way of sharing the good news that men and women do not have to merely yield to diabetes in middle age.

The dietary battle wouldn't be nearly so difficult if so many Americans did not eat so poorly. Though you aren't a freak, you will at times *feel* like one, so different will be your way of eating. You will find encouragement in these two things:

- First, *there are so many low-carb substitutes and snacks that you are not giving up nearly so much as you might suppose.* I hear things like, "I don't think I could ever give up cake, or candy, or potatoes, or..." People say, "I would feel so cheated..." The truth is, I don't feel cheated at all. I feel blessed. I value my health far above any culinary delights. I thank God continually for delivering me from diabetes. He hasn't cheated me; He has blessed me incredibly. I have been "deprived" of insulin shots, blindness, amputations, and early death.

- *Second, you will simply be doing what you need to do.* In my case, I should have been far more moderate in my use of sugar and refined flour in my earlier years. If I had, I might not need to take the steps I am taking today. But in any case, the Creator provides me so many pleasures in life that far exceed food. Playing golf with my sons, praying in the early morning and sensing the sweetness of the Holy Spirit's presence as He prepares me for the day ahead, finding a good deal at a garage sale, holding my new granddaughter—life is good because God is good.

To give up a slice of sugar-laden chocolate cake is nothing. (Plus, I still can enjoy low-carb desserts that taste every bit as good to me as their carb-laden cousins.)

The Second Front: Exercise

The second front of your war for the health of your body is the area of exercise. While I acknowledge diet as the most important front, this does not mean that exercise is merely optional. Exercise is a must for everyone who is serious about attaining optimal health. Not only will physical inactivity shorten your life; it will make the years you do have less pleasant and more troublesome.

Keep in mind that we are not talking about turning everybody into a world-class athlete. It is not necessary that you run windsprints for an hour a day, or develop muscles like a bodybuilder, or attain the stamina of a marathoner. (It is advisable, though, to check with your doctor before beginning an exercise program.)

A brisk walk or a light jog four to five times a week for 30 to 40 minutes a session is enough. The exercise does not have to be extremely painful or wear you out so you are worthless for the next three hours. Almost anyone can do the kinds of exercise needful for maintaining a healthy metabolism.

In preparing for this, there are two important areas of consideration. First, you will need, if at all possible, to invest in a piece of exercise equipment. For my money, a good treadmill is your best choice. It can be argued that it is healthier to walk outdoors than to do a treadmill indoors. And that is probably true. The problem is, setting up for a walk or jog outdoors is more complicated than indoor exercise. In most parts of the country weather becomes a factor. There is nothing inherently evil about walking or jogging in the rain, but most of us won't do it. During the winter, cold weather either stops us from exercise or else adds another negative factor that makes it easier to miss a day here and there. In the summer, it is often so hot that the jog or walk seems easier to miss than to do.

Making It Regular

Second, the biggest part of exercise is simply the discipline to do it regularly. Any factor which will increase that likelihood is to be strongly desired. Here is where a treadmill excels. Mainly, you decrease the amount of time involved. At one point in my life I lived a couple of minutes away from a beautiful park which had a concrete jogging and walking path that wove around a lake. It was scenic and a great place for me to jog. However, even with the track that close and the beauty of the park, I still was not able to be as consistent as I needed to be. Just the act of getting into my car and going to the park took time and created one extra small psychological hurdle. At times the rain kept me from jogging. At other times, after a big rain, the track would be so littered with debris and mud I would skip several days until things dried up.

Heat in the summer would sometimes keep me at home. And as pretty as the park was, there was the monotony of going around that same track, time after time, with nothing to do but think. The park was a blessing—but it wasn't until I got a treadmill, along with a big hypogly-cemic scare, that I was able to attain real consistency in exercise.

I "treat" myself now when I exercise on the treadmill—by taping History Channel documentaries in advance and then watching them as I exercise. I even have head-phones hooked up so I can hear better and don't have to blast the entire family out of the house to be able to hear over the treadmill. When I tape a really juicy docu-mentary, like a two-hour special about the last year of the Civil War or the story of the creation of the atomic bomb, I can hardly wait to exercise again so I can see them.

As a result of this, plus the fact that I nearly always do my exercising in the morning, I am usually able to get in five or six days a week. (I never do seven, believing that God had His reasons for commanding us to observe a day of rest each week.) In sum, purchasing a treadmill, or some other aerobic machine is one of the best invest-ments you can make to ensure a well-oiled metabolism. If you can't afford a new one, go to garage sales. You won't be at many before you find one—usually for about $50. If even that is too much, there is always the old-fashioned exercise called outdoor walking. Just be sure to have a contingency plan for days that are too cold, too hot, too rainy, or any other "too's" your mind can come up with. Go up and down your stairs for a half hour or use a stepper with a video if necessary.

The key thing is to make sure you are exercising more days per week than not. Plan ahead for success. Most of you reading this book can scrape together enough cash over a month or two to purchase at least a used treadmill, rowing machine, or some other piece of aerobic exercise equipment. Go for it! This equipment will be a friend for life (yours or its). Regular use could easily improve your fasting blood sugar by ten points or more, and could take you from diabetic to borderline, or from borderline to normal. Combined with a low-carb diet and a normal weight, your blood-sugar woes could be over forever! These measures are a tiny price to pay to have your health back.

The Third Front: Weight

For many of you, the third front is the scariest of all. You may already be saying, "I might be able to handle the change of food, and I'm game to attempt regular exercise, but don't ask me to do anything about my weight. I've already 'been there, done that.' I just can't lose weight."

Well, as a matter of fact, weight may be the easiest battlefront of all. The reason is this: If you change to a low-carb diet and begin to exercise regularly, you will almost automatically begin to lose weight, especially if you are overweight by more than 40 pounds. The late Dr. Atkins and other low-carb gurus originally got into the low-carb lifestyle as a means of losing weight, and only later realized what tremendous health benefits there were from this more natural way of eating.

But as with the other two fronts of your battle to regain healthy blood-sugar levels, you must have a plan. You cannot amble into permanent weight loss; you must charge in with a plan and the determination that comes from knowing your plan is sound and victory is attainable.

As with exercise, you need to make a small financial investment. Purchase the best digital scale you can afford. You will need to weigh yourself every day in order to get the feedback that serves as such a wonderful motivator. Negative behaviors (along with cockroaches) always flourish best in darkness. As long as you don't think much about weight, don't measure your progress (or the lack thereof), you will be unsuccessful in any attempt to lose weight. You are going to have to determine an optimal weight for yourself and begin to move toward that goal.

In the chapter on weight loss I will go into more specific ways you can do this, but again, you must keep in mind that the patterns you establish will need to be lifetime habits. You are not going on a "diet." You are not going to sprint your way to the desired weight. (There is such a thing as losing weight too fast. Not only is this not good for your health, it is actually conducive to regaining the weight you just lost.) Your weight loss must be *gradual, purposeful, and permanent.*

Encouragement As You Prepare

You can win. Too many people have simply given up after multiple fad diets and false starts. You can win through the knowledge that arriving at the proper weight is not merely for the sake of looking better and impressing your friends; it is the best way to take care of the body the Creator has entrusted to you.

You must win. As long as you are overweight, you are straining every system in your body. This is especially true of your metabolic system. The fat that accumulates around your waistline and on your arms and legs is notoriously inefficient at handling sugar. It doesn't just look bad; it's killing you. Losing weight is not an option anymore.

Think About It!

One of the most important things you can do in preparation for the battles on the fronts of diet, exercise, and weight is simply to think about them. Pray about them. As you think and pray, you will be conditioning yourself to win. Spend a little cash to provide the equipment that will help you in your path to victory.

Any pattern of living which is ruinous to our health is an area that must be dealt with. You are too valuable to exit the stage early in the play. As Jimmy Stewart found out, it really is a wonderful life, and there are lots of people depending upon you.

CHAPTER 7

The First Front: Diet Deletions

⟶

Unless you have been sleeping while reading the earlier chapters of this book (a pretty neat trick) you will have already figured out that I am going to be talking about a low-carb diet. The most famous proponent of low-carb eating was the late Dr. Atkins, who primarily touted this diet for weight loss, but also demonstrated several other health benefits of it.

Almost everyone agrees that low-carb eating is effective in promoting weight loss. Where the argument gets hot and heavy is in whether such a diet is actually good for you. Many proclaim that eating unlimited meat and cheese will raise your cholesterol levels out of sight and bring you to an early death as a result of heart failure. You will lose weight and make a skinny corpse!

Atkins started touting low-carb eating in the 1970s and was immediately branded a dietary heretic, a wacky far-out nut no sensible person would heed. Amazingly he would not go away. And the more he preached, the more people listened, and results almost always followed. Finally the medical establishment had no choice but to investigate. In the last few years several serious studies have been done and, to everyone's astonishment, they all demonstrate positive results for the Atkins approach. Not only do people lose weight more effectively on a low-carb diet, their triglycerides (a major sign of potential heart disease) decrease, and their total cholesterol either stays the same, or, in many cases, is significantly lowered.

In one recent study, it was found that people who went on the traditional low-fat, high-carb diet decreased their triglycerides by 1 percent, whereas those on the low-carb diet decreased their triglycerides by 28 percent. (Triglycerides measure the fat in the bloodstream.) One would logically think that the more fat you eat, the higher your blood fats would rise, and by eating less fat, you would achieve lower blood fat. It seems to make sense, but the body doesn't work that way. That common assumption ignores the powerful role of excess insulin in raising blood fats and cholesterol.

Rather, reductions in triglycerides, as well as cholesterol and blood-sugar, are the rule and not the exception when a high-carb, high-sugar diet is replaced with a high-protein, low-carb regimen.

A Lifesaving Decrease

In the book *Protein Power,* Dr. Michael Eades tells of one of his patients. Jane came to him with cholesterol and tryglyceride levels that were nearly off the charts. Her tryglyceride levels measured at a life-threatening 495 mg/dl. Her blood sugar was at the diabetic level of 155 mg/dl. After Eades took her off her cholesterol-lowering medication, put her on a diet that allowed red meat, cheese, eggs, and other "no-no's," and told her to reduce her carb intake, she returned to the office in six weeks with some pretty miraculous results. Her cholesterol took a nose-dive from 495 to 186. Her triglycerides went from 495 to 86 md/dl. Her blood sugar went from a diabetic 155 to a perfectly normal (even better than normal) 86 mg/dl.[1]

Nobody expected this. The only knock left on Atkins at this point is that these studies were short-term, and "we'll have to wait and see what the long-term results are."

The central truth these studies are demonstrating is something almost no nutritionist realized: The amount of cholesterol you put in your mouth has very little to do with the amount of cholesterol that accumulates in your body. A jelly doughnut may be far more harmful to your heart than a steak! The key is insulin production.

Let's consider the notorious egg. It is a well-known fact that an egg, ounce for ounce, is loaded with cholesterol. Nutritionists and doctors naturally assumed that the more eggs you eat, the higher your cholesterol level will rise. For this reason, people who have had heart attacks or bypasses, or whose cholesterol level was unacceptably high, have been told to swear off eggs completely.

It sounds reasonable. You take in more cholesterol, and your body stores up more cholesterol. The problem is, studies do not bear this out. An article written in the *New England Journal of Medicine* startled the medical community when it revealed that a man who had been in the habit of eating 25 eggs a day for the last 30 years had normal cholesterol levels.[2] Why wasn't all the cholesterol from all those eggs simply adding up in his body to produce towering cholesterol levels? (Or, more to our point, why was this man still alive?)

A Clear Phenomenon

Eskimos have traditionally lived on a high-fat, very-low-carb diet. According to the popular theory of nutrition, they should lead the world in heart disease. In fact, they suffer very little from heart problems, obesity, blood-pressure problems, or diabetes. For a meat-eating, fat-consuming, bagel-less people, they are remarkably healthy.

In the 1920s Arctic explorer Vilhjalmur Stefansson went an entire year eating nothing but fresh fish and meat and drinking only water. Amazingly not only did he not get scurvy, but at the end of the period his cholesterol counts were lower than they were at the beginning.[3]

In the 1960s Dr. Anatolio Cruz oversaw an experiment revealing the effect of excess insulin upon arteries. His team injected insulin into the large arteries of one of the legs of dogs. The other was injected with saline. After eight months the effects of the insulin were pronounced: The arteries injected with it had a high degree of accumulated cholesterol and fatty acids, with the inner arterial lining considerably thickened. The arteries injected with saline remained normal.[4]

Studies strongly suggest our problems with heart disease and blood-sugar control have far more to do with the amount of excess insulin our overworked pancreas must produce than the amount of cholesterol in the steaks, eggs, and cheese we eat. In our attempts to "eat healthy" we have cut back on the steaks and filled ourselves with breads and sugars.

While we could get away with this in our youth, by the time we hit our late 40s or early 50s (sometimes well before) our weakened metabolism cannot keep up the pace. Though our blood sugar may not be fully out of control at diabetic levels, it is taking more and more insulin to keep our blood sugar at a normal level. As we discussed in chapter 3, our overworked pancreas gamely pumps out huge amounts of insulin just trying to keep up with all the sugars and starches we are ingesting. As a result we are doing to ourselves what Dr. Anatolio Cruz did to the dogs he experimented with (see sidebar beginning on the previous page). We are overloading our bodies with insulin. Heart disease and diabetes, those twin diseases of "civilization," are the tragic result. Dr. Michael Eades sums it up thus:

In the appropriate amount insulin keeps the metabolic system humming along smoothly with everything in balance; in great excess it becomes a rogue hormone raging throughout the body, wreaking metabolic havoc, and leaving a trail of chaos and disease in its wake.[5]

How I Differ from Dr. Atkins

While the diet I am recommending to you is similar to the one Dr. Atkins espoused, there are a few differences. Atkins was a purist; I am not. He also had strong opinions on almost all types of foods; I will concern myself with what you need to achieve healthy blood-sugar levels and be kind to your pancreas. (I like that expression. Maybe we need a national "Be Kind to Your Pancreas Day"!)

A few examples. Atkins frowns on caffeine. He states that it may actually lower blood-sugar levels, but for any but a coffee fanatic, a couple of cups of coffee or tea each day will have almost no effect upon blood sugar one way or another. (If you load your coffee with sugary creamers and then top it with a couple of heaping teaspoons of sugar, that's a different story of course!) Atkins is probably right that we might be better off if we totally forgot about coffee and tea, but when we are attempting to make the necessary sacrifices to corral our runaway blood sugars, the last thing we need to do is make an issue of peripherals that really don't make that much difference. There are enough real sacrifices you will need to make—without adding nonessentials to the list.

Another example is aspartame. Atkins doesn't like aspartame and recommends Splenda. I use Splenda as a substitute sweetener when possible, but there are too many good products that use aspartame for me to give it up entirely. Almost every diet soda is sweetened by aspartame. One of the keys to staying with a diet for the long haul (as in "your whole life") is making it as "pain free" as possible. By replacing regular sodas with aspartame-sweetened sodas (which contain no carbs at all) you don't have to feel like you are being left out altogether. I certainly don't recommend drinking eight or ten diet Cokes a day, but having a diet soda every other day or so is no big deal. It will have little effect upon your blood sugars, and it makes a great drink to go with your taco (made with a low-carb tortilla shell) or your snack of peanuts.

Another beef (no pun intended!) I have with Atkins and some other proponents of low-carb eating has to do with the sample menus they list. It's not that the recipes they provide don't fit the low-carb pattern. They certainly do. But they are often not for people who live in the real world. One of Atkins' recipes calls for a pound of cleaned squid. Cleaned squid! Where do you get cleaned squid (or dirty squid for that matter)? While Atkins does give many recipes with more common ingredients, they usually contain a great many spices and unusual ingredients that are costly and time-consuming to track down and purchase. Reading these recipes can get a little depressing. You get the impression that to do the low-carb diet you have to become the Galloping Gourmet (for you younger folks, he was a well-known TV chef in ancient days)!

The truth is, there are lots of ways of using basic foods that don't cost a lot or require an advanced degree in kitchenology for you to prepare. Anyone with the desire to eat healthy and a little know-how can start enjoying a low-carb cuisine immediately. Part of the secret is in knowing what not to eat; the other part is in having a ready supply of foods and snacks that are blood-sugar friendly.

What a Low-Carb Diet Is *Not* (Dispelling the Myths)

When you mention a low-carb diet to many people, their first thought is of somebody stuffing themselves with sausages, steaks, and eggs, never eating any vegetables or fruits, sending their cholesterol levels sky-high, and coming down with scurvy and rickets for the lack of vitamins. On top of that they expect low-carbers to be in a constant state of constipation for lack of fiber. Such is far from the case.

Going low-carb does not mean that you live on meat and eggs and avoid anything that might have vitamins in it. Keep in mind that low-carb is not no-carb. It would be folly to suggest we are supposed to do away with all carbohydrates and live on meat alone. The truth is, there are plenty of people who have never considered a low-carb lifestyle and eat far more meat than I do. As I came to understand that our greatest dietary problem is our overconsumption of carbohydrates and not the eating of meat, I became much less fearful of meat. I no longer ruin my steak dinners with guilty thoughts of clogging my arteries with plaque. As long as I avoid the rolls, doughnuts, and Snickers bars, the cholesterol in the meat is going to pass right on through.

Now, allow me to introduce to you God's gracious gift to healthy eaters—the salad. While salad does indeed contain carbohydrates, these carbohydrates come in the best possible form. Most of the ingredients in a typical salad—lettuce, radishes, broccoli, cauliflower, and so forth—are fairly low in carbs, and the carbs they do have are locked into their fibers so they are released slowly into the bloodstream. As a result they are a kinder, gentler form of carbs, which our pancreas can easily handle. Such a salad is filled with vitamins, has lots of fiber, and is a wonderful complement to your meat dish.

Since going low-carb I have eaten more salads than I ever have in my life, and I would expect I eat more salad than the vast majority of people who eat traditional American fare. I do not sit down to a dinner of huge steaks, followed by quarter-pound burgers topped with pounds of bacon and a half-dozen eggs. If you didn't watch carefully you might not even notice that my meal was low-carb, it would look so normal.

An example of a typical meal for me might include a salmon patty, a large salad, and a low-carb muffin. If I am extra hungry that night I might also have a celery stalk filled with peanut butter. I leave the table filled and feeling great in the knowledge I have not pushed my pancreas to the limit. (As I mentioned, I know it is not necessary for me to take a blood-sugar reading after such a meal. I have taken enough readings to know that this kind of meal will leave my blood-sugar levels low and will help ensure that my pancreas continues to do its important job for years to come.) Every such meal keeps the terrible specter of diabetes at bay. String together enough of these kinds of meals (about 40 years' worth or so, if you are middle-aged) and you will probably enjoy a lifetime of blood-sugar health. In the process you will do a lot for your heart as well.

The No-No's and the Maybe So's

I've said it before but I'll say it again—there *are* some sacrifices to be made. While there are some wonderful substitutes for many foods, there's no getting around the fact that if you are to get serious about your blood sugar, you are going to have to give up some pretty great-tasting foods. Let's look at some of them.

The Potato

The potato is a wonderful food in many respects. It can be cooked in a myriad of ways, it tastes great in almost every way you can think to cook it, it is relatively nutritious, and it makes a wonderful side dish. It is also murder on those who have blood-sugar difficulties. While you may get by with having a small amount of potatoes occasionally, for the most part you are going to have to say goodbye to Mr. Potato.

The reason is this: Potatoes are about as starchy a food as you can find on planet Earth. They quickly turn into sugar in your bloodstream. Eating a large baked potato is as taxing on your pancreas and insulin receptors as a Snickers candy bar. While the sugar doesn't hit your system quite as fast, it doesn't take long for that starchy potato to turn into sugar and drive your pancreas crazy.

You may argue, "But a potato is so natural! How can it be bad for you?" It isn't bad for everyone. People whose blood-sugar mechanisms are humming along beautifully can eat them with no problem. And if you had been more discriminating in weight control, diet, and exercise in your last 30 or 40 years, you might be able to eat potatoes every day for the rest of your life and be fine. But that is not how things are. The fact that you are reading this book indicates that you most likely have done some permanent damage to your body, and can no longer endure a food that, other than its starchiness, is fantastic.

In a way your situation is like the alcoholic who, out of desperation, gives up every trace of alcohol for the rest of his days. He goes out to dinner with a friend, who casually orders a glass of wine. While his friend can drink the wine without the slightest temptation to "go on a binge," the alcoholic cannot. He must, for reasons that don't seem quite fair, give up that which others don't need to. So it is with the glorious potato. *Au revoir, hasta luego, sayonara, arrivederci*...however you choose to say it, you and Mr. Potato are going to have to part company if you are serious about your blood-sugar levels.

Doing away with potatoes is actually more of a pain than the fact that we lost a tasty friend. The potato plays a major role as a side dish in so many of our meals. Spaghetti and hash browns, hamburgers and french fries, stroganoff and baked potatoes, pork chops and fried potatoes...well, you get the idea. If you deduct the potato from meals, it is a crisis of major proportions. How in the world will we ever get full?

As you grow in your knowledge of nutrition and pancreas-friendly foods, you will discover your own personal preferences for potato substitutes. For dinner I almost always enjoy a large salad as my potato substitute. Sometimes I will have a good sized helping of cooked cauliflower covered with melted cheese. A Wasa cracker (see page 116) covered with cream cheese will work, as will a helping of cottage cheese and berries (unsweetened). Celery with peanut butter is filling and delicious. There are ways to get around it, but I will be the first to admit that I sometimes miss my friend, Mr. Potato. But he's not such a good friend that I would trade my health and shorten my life just to keep his company!

Rice

Rice, like the potato, is a starch which turns into sugar in your bloodstream. It is not as bad an offender as the potato, but it is not a food which you will want to eat frequently. Those times when you do eat rice, make sure that it is brown, whole-grain rice. This rice is still a high-carb food, but it, like all whole-grain products, releases its carbs slower than its white brother and produces less strain on your blood-sugar system. I occasionally have a dinner in which rice plays a part, but I make sure to take a smaller portion of the rice and make up for it by taking bigger portions of the low-carb foods. Except in emergency situations, people with blood-sugar problems should leave white rice alone and limit their consumption of brown rice to infrequent occasions, taking small portions when they do indulge.

Beans

Beans are another high-carb food that seem to be innocuous. They are high in fiber, have more protein than most non-meat foods, and are considered healthy by almost everybody. Truth is beans are great—for those without blood-sugar difficulties. For you who are reading this book, beans are not the best of foods. Because they are high in fiber and release their carbs more slowly, they are definitely a better choice than the potato. A small helping of beans is usually not a big deal. But a large helping, such as a large bowl of bean soup, will definitely raise your blood-sugar levels. It will take longer than a candy bar or orange juice, but when the beans begin to break down in your stomach, your pancreas will know it. Beans sweetened with brown sugar or corn syrup are a double curse. Stay away!

Fruits

"Surely you wouldn't ask me to give up fruit! Why fruit is so...natural!" Fruit is natural, but what is not natural is how much of it we eat and how constantly we eat it. In nature fruit comes in season for a very brief period. During that time, our ancestors would enjoy their peaches, or apples, or whatever. But when that brief period of ripeness was over, they would say goodbye to that fruit for about a year. Today, when you have two or three fruits a day, all year long, along with sodas, desserts, and mountains of white bread and pasta, it is simply too much.

Make no mistake. Fruit is far superior to candy or pie. The sugars that most fruits carry are locked in fiber, which makes them easier to handle. But people with runaway blood sugar cannot indulge in fruit whenever they like and however much they want. There is a good reason why people like them so much. Most of them are quite high in sugar content. And even "natural" sugars will take their toll on you. (God explicitly gives us wisdom on this in Proverbs 25:16: "Have you found honey? Eat only as much as you need, lest you be filled with it and vomit.")

Not all fruits are created alike. Be a discriminating fruit connoisseur. The worst form of fruit is fruit juice. In this way you are getting the natural sugars without their natural houses—fiber. Many fruit juices are every bit as sweet as soda, and should be avoided at all times. (The banana is a good example of a fruit that would surprise most people—see sidebar.)

Don't Go Bananas!

Bananas don't seem all that sweet, and everyone knows they are loaded with potassium and other good stuff. Surely the banana is okay.

Not really. I learned this in my early days, when I was testing nearly every meal with my glucometer about an hour after I ate. I had just eaten what I thought was a great low-carb meal of salmon, a salad, some other small dish, and a banana. When I took my blood sugar I expected a great reading and

was dismayed when my reading turned out somewhere around 150. I was so shocked I did some investigating and finally discovered that the banana was
the offending food. A large banana can have over 30
grams of carbs in it—about the same amount as you
would find in a candy bar! I might as well have had
a Three Musketeers bar as far as my blood sugar was
concerned.

I rarely eat bananas today. I know they are
a great source of potassium, but they are not the
only source of potassium. Cows and penguins and
lions get potassium in other ways and have strong,
healthy bodies without ever touching bananas. So
can you. If you are determined to eat bananas, never
eat a whole one. Have them a half at a time, and
find somebody else to give the other half to. If, after
your meal with your half-banana, your blood sugar
is in good order, fine. If not, you may need to hold a
funeral for the nice but naughty banana.

The fruits most acceptable for blood-sugar-challenged
folks like us are the berries. Strawberries, raspberries, blue-
berries, and blackberries are sweet but not all that sweet.
They are great over a small bowl of cottage cheese (far
superior to the standard canned peaches in heavy syrup!).
Just be sure that you buy berries that have not been sweetened. Berries can also make a great topping on the dozens
of the low-carb cheesecakes you can find recipes for on
the Internet.

102 OVERCOMING RUNAWAY BLOOD SUGAR

Sweets

By sweets I simply mean all those desserts, candies, ice-cream bars, and other "foods" that are essentially an excuse for you to fill your body with sugar. Often people writing about diabetes try to soft-pedal the issue of sweets by saying that you can still eat these scrumptious treats; you just have to count your carbs. It gives me the picture of someone who eats no carbs all day long—and then at nine in the evening stuffs himself with a huge piece of apple pie smothered in ice cream. Sorry, folks—it ain't gonna work!

The only reason I can see for ever having any of these blood-sugar disturbers is if your willpower is such that you feel you would never be able to maintain a low-carb diet without occasionally "cheating." If that is truly the case, then go ahead and splurge once in a while, but do it by plan, not by yielding to the desire of the moment. And make sure and have the smallest helping you can possibly have for your yielding to be worthwhile.

Actually there really is no reason to have normal "sweets" these days, because there are so many low-carb substitutes available. When I first figured out what I needed to do to get control of my blood sugar, one of the biggest sacrifices for me was my evening routine. For years my wife and I were in the habit of ending our evenings by watching something on TV and having a snack with coffee. (For some reason neither of us had any trouble sleeping after a cup of coffee.) We would have some pretty incredible (but intense) sweets to go with our evening coffee: homemade cinnamon rolls, coconut pies, brownies, and all sorts of other fattening, high-carb goodies.

After going low-carb I didn't know what I was going to do. Being a man who loves routines and rituals, it was unthinkable to give up the evening coffee and snack. But what to eat? At first I started with cottage cheese and a couple of slices of peaches (from fresh peaches, not the syrupy stuff you find in cans). But somehow cottage cheese and peaches just seemed a pretty wimpy snack to eat while I sipped my coffee and watched *Andy Griffith* reruns.

As my eyes opened to the tremendous varieties of low-carb foods and snacks available on the grocery shelves and through low-carb companies, my choices suddenly mushroomed. Low-carb bars and low-carb brownies went a whole lot better with the coffee than the cottage cheese had. And then one day I got on the Internet and typed "low-carb recipes" on a search engine. Immediately I came up with enough sites and recipes to last me for a dozen lifetimes. Some of these desserts are every bit as good as the high-carb pies and treats I had eaten before. The difference is that with the previous snacks I was forcing my blood-sugar system to deal with 50 to 70 grams of carbs; now I was enjoying snacks that added a mere 5 to 10 grams of carbs. My pancreas thanked me, my insulin receptor cells thanked me, and we were all happy. Even friends and family who don't struggle with blood-sugar issues have had to admit that some of these desserts are really good.

At the writing of this book I am 50 years of age. If the Lord grants that I live to the average age expectancy of 76 years, I have about 26 more years of low-carb eating. Because of the wonderful substitutes available, I am not making nearly the sacrifice I would otherwise have to. I can handle low-carb eating for 26 more years. It's a price I will gladly pay for my health!

Pasta

Next to potatoes, pasta is the product which most Americans will have a hard time doing without. We use pasta in so many of our foods. Spaghetti, casseroles of all kinds, beef stroganoff... Americans love their pasta. In with the low-fat, high-carb diet, we have actually been told that pasta is good for us. Athletes are told to load up on the pasta for greater strength and endurance.

The truth is, pasta is an unnatural food which is made of refined flour and drives blood-sugar levels berserk in susceptible people. It has very little nutritional value, very little fiber, tends to clog up our colons, and is mostly a filler. You are doing yourself no favor by eating lots of pasta.

There are pasta substitutes. These low-carb pastas use a lot of soy, and usually have about a third of the carbs of regular pasta. There is a problem, however. To be honest, many of these pastas simply don't taste very good. And some of them taste absolutely terrible. I suffered through some of these pastas until I discovered the wonderful spaghetti squash. This squash has what looks pretty much like noodles inside it, and these taste great with spaghetti sauce over them. Spaghetti night is no longer a problem for me.

If you are serious about wanting to get your blood sugar under control naturally, you will need to permanently forsake regular pasta. It has little nutrition, little fiber, and will drive your blood-sugar levels crazy.

At times you may be with a crowd who decides to

go to an Italian or other all-pasta restaurant. In some of these places it is almost impossible to find a main dish that doesn't include lots of pasta. I try to avoid them at all costs, but if I am forced into such a place, I'll go with the chef salad, which almost every restaurant has. It may not be as filling as a huge plateful of lasagna, but I'll leave knowing that my blood sugar has not skyrocketed. And that's a great feeling!

Bread

Here's a surprise for you. Bread, by the slice, isn't really that bad of a food, carb-wise. Now, before you fall into a faint, let me explain. A slice of whole-wheat bread (at least the kind that I buy) has 11 grams per slice. But it has 3 grams of fiber, which can be deducted from the total, since fiber doesn't affect blood sugar. So when you eat a slice of bread you are only ingesting 8 grams of carbs. That's really not too bad, as long as you don't get too many carbs from other sources.

You can put lots of different kinds of meats and cheeses on a slice of bread and make a pretty filling sandwich (leave off the top piece, preferably). Even two slices of bread, 16 grams of carbs, is probably okay at a meal, *as long as you stay away from other major sources of carbs.* In other words, don't have a meal that includes bread and rice, or bread and pasta, or bread and potatoes. As an afternoon snack I often have a piece of bread with peanut butter on it. People seeing me eat it and knowing that I am on a low-carb diet would think me a hypocrite or a weakling, but it is all part of the schedule. It is far superior to a piece of cake, a bowl of cereal, or milk and cookies.

The Nature's Own brand has come out with a low-carb bread that can be bought at many grocery stores. This bread, after fiber is deducted, is only five carbs, which is better still. You can even enjoy a sandwich with top and bottom slices. Sometimes I have a peanut butter and jelly sandwich with this kind of bread. Because the jelly is low-carb jelly (about one gram per tablespoon) and the bread is low-carb bread, I am actually eating a low-carb food! It's amazing how good we have it today!

This having been said, you must be careful to avoid things like doughnuts (ugh) and bagels (often containing as many as 50 grams of carbs each—try Atkins brand low-carb bagels, which are surprisingly good), rolls and biscuits, and all other sorts of white bread products. Sometimes at our Friday morning prayer breakfast I do allow myself a half biscuit with gravy. By loading up on the eggs and bacon, the half biscuit satisfies me, and I don't feel cheated. I checked my blood sugar after such a meal and found that my system can handle it without any significant rise in blood sugar. But if I were to eat like the old Dennis sometimes did—eating two or three biscuits, some with gravy and some with jelly, I would be overloading my system and creating major havoc for my body.

I am 50; I am not 20 and I'm not 30. I simply cannot do what I once could. It wasn't good for me to eat that way then, and it would be far worse for me to try to eat like that now. I have lived what was probably the first two-thirds of my life eating for my own pleasure; this last third (the Lord willing) I will eat for my health and His glory.

The thing that saddens me and even amazes me is to see men who are full-fledged diabetics ingesting large amounts of carbs at every meal. I suppose they reason that they can just take a pill or give themselves a shot, and all will be well. This kind of thinking leads to the progressive worsening of their condition and eventually results in miseries of all kinds, including amputations and premature death. The Bible says that the prudent man sees evil coming and hides himself (Proverbs 22:3). There are a lot of diabetics around that have never learned that simple lesson. One of the great tragedies of diabetes is that with a few basic lifestyle changes many that are on insulin could be on pills, and many that are on pills could be off medication altogether. And nearly all could live healthier, longer lives.

Milk

I hate to tell you this, but milk is a fairly high-carb drink. An eight-ounce glass of milk has 12 grams of carbs in it. Now, if this was your only source of carbs for your meal, it wouldn't be too bad, but considering that most meals are going to include some carbs from other sources, it doesn't make sense to add an extra 12 grams to each meal simply for the luxury of a glass of milk. This is especially true with cereal, which will have lots of carbs already. Add an extra 12 grams to the 40 or 50 grams that the cereal provides and you are getting as many carbs as if you ate almost two candy bars. Even the whole-grain cereals can play havoc on your blood-sugar levels, so you're going to need to give up that bowl-of-raisin-bran breakfast. (I am a cereal lover. Giving up cereal was one of my greatest sacrifices. But as John Wayne would have said, "A man's gotta do what a man's gotta do!")

By the way, you need to be careful in reading labels.

When you look at a box of cereal you can easily be misled. For example, Kellogg's Raisin Bran lists its nutrition facts for a serving size of one cup: 45 grams. But did you ever measure out one cup of cereal? It is exceedingly tiny. Almost nobody would eat such a small amount. In the real world, most of us would eat at least two cups, and big eaters would probably eat three. Two cups of raisin bran would be 90 carbs, the milk would add an extra 12 carbs, so that you are getting more than 100 grams of carbs from a single bowl of cereal. You can deduct 14 grams for the fiber, but you are still getting an enormous load of carbs for your blood-sugar system to deal with, and usually at the worst possible time. Our metabolism is at its worst in the morning, due to the fact that we haven't been active for about eight hours or longer. Having a bowl of raisin bran is the blood-sugar equivalent of having two-and-a-half candy bars for breakfast. For people with blood-sugar problems, it is the height of folly to eat such a breakfast. By the way, I'm only using raisin bran as an example because most people would consider this the ideal "healthy" cereal, being made with whole grains and containing raisins (sugar-coated ones). Trix, Cap'n Crunch, and the rest of the gang are that much worse!

I have hit only the major sources of carbs. There are others, but you will need to do a little investigating on your own. Let's go to a new chapter and talk about the good stuff now!

CHAPTER 8

The First Front: Diet Additions

Study after study of low-carb dieting indicates that high cholesterol levels are a result of the high-carb diet, as we've seen. Such a diet provokes a flood of insulin into the bloodstream, especially as people reach middle age and become more insulin-resistant. The more insulin-resistant you become, the more insulin your pancreas is forced to release to deal with blood sugar. Even though your blood-sugar levels may not be all that high, your body is producing enormous amounts of insulin to do what a tiny little squirt would manage 20 years earlier.

There is so much you can do about this, however. And the great thing is, much of the food you will need to center your diet on is just plain good stuff! This chapter will give you some whats, hows, and whys.

Meat

The medical establishment and nutritional gurus have done their best to turn Americans from their love affair with meat, and if not stopping us altogether, at least making us feel guilty when we do indulge.

But for people with blood-sugar woes, meat is a trusty friend. It is filling, tastes great, and barely affects your blood sugar. When I have a meal with a large steak or hamburger patty, I know that I'm going to get filled, and do my body no harm. And while that steak contains a great deal more cholesterol than a tofu sandwich, as long as I keep my insulin level low by not challenging my blood-sugar level with mega doses of carbs, that cholesterol is going to pass right on through.

It would be foolish to read this book and immediately go to stuffing yourself with meat at every available opportunity—huge amounts of bacon and sausage for breakfast, a couple of quarter-pounders for lunch, an enormous steak for dinner, and a midnight snack of several pounds of ribs. Meat is not the ogre that overzealous nutritionists have made it out to be, but like everything else, it should be eaten in moderation. Man does not live by bread alone (especially the diabetic), and it is likewise true that we should not live on meat alone either.

Be sure and eat good supplies of fish and fowl, along with red meat and pork. Red meat is not as bad as some claim, but you will do better to eat a variety of meat, and especially to include fish in your diet.

Salad

We have already talked about salad, but I can't help but give a little more testimony to this wonderful friend of those who struggle with blood-sugar control. The salad will be a major side dish (and sometimes main dish) for the rest of your life. Experiment with different types of salads (stay away from Mexican salads—taco salads—with the beans and chips), and learn to look on them as most people see potatoes!

Salads do have carbs, but they don't have a lot of carbs. And the carbs that they do have are released slowly into your bloodstream, due to the fact that they are locked in roughage. While most people consider the potato their main secondary item after a meat or pasta dish, you should consider the salad to fulfill this role. Find several low-carb salad dressings you like (avoid french and thousand island for sure!) and indulge.

While a meat-only diet would be high in protein but sadly deficient in roughage and vitamins, your friendly salad makes up for these. Don't just make your salad with lettuce and tomatoes. Be creative. Vary your salads, but use lots of ingredients such as cucumbers, radishes, broccoli, cauliflower, green peppers, and so forth. Because carrots are one of the vegetables highest in sugar content, you will want to go easy on them, but a few slices of carrot will do you no harm.

Because I eat very little fruit anymore, I make up for this by eating far more salads than before. Most people's idea of a low-carb diet is constantly stuffing yourself with steak and eggs, and eating little else. Let them follow me around for a few days. They will find that I eat more vegetables than most Americans, and get them in the healthier, uncooked form. Because the low-carb diet makes weight control almost irrelevant (you will find it almost impossible to get and stay overweight if you stick with this diet), I can enjoy a regular salad dressing without concern. Those low fat dressings leave a lot to be desired. Since I do sacrifice certain foods and culinary pleasures, it is nice to be able to indulge in a great tasting dressing!

Nuts!

This was the famous reply given by Brigadier General Anthony McAuliffe at Bastogne during the Battle of the Bulge when the Americans were surrounded and asked by the Germans if they were ready to surrender. (I threw that in for all the history buffs.) Nuts are a great source of protein and a low-carb food that goes with nearly every-thing. Being a nut lover anyway, no one has to twist my arm to eat nuts. While nuts are high in fats and high in protein, they are relatively low in carbs. Another wonderful feature about most nuts is that they have one of the lowest ratings of any foods on the glycemic index.

What Is the Glycemic Index?

The glycemic index is a rating system given to foods that ranks how easily and quickly their carbs turn into sugars in your bloodstream. We are not talking about the amount of carbs, but simply how fast they break down into sugar; in other words how much stress they put on your pancreas after eating them.

> Obviously the foods that are best for you are those foods which break down very slowly and gradually in your system. The scale runs from 1 to 100, with the foods which break down quickest at the high end. Thus a baked potato ranks up there at 85, while a bowl of All-Bran cereal is much lower at 42.

For instance, can you guess the ranking of the lowly peanut? The peanut comes in at an incredible 14. There is hardly a food which ranks any better. When you combine the lower amount of carbs in nuts, along with the very slow release of their carbs into glucose, you have a great food. Peanuts can be that extra food you need to fill up, when you still feel hungry at the end of your meal. They can be substituted for potatoes, and taste great in balancing the sweetness of a low-carb bar. One caution: If you're going to eat a lot of nuts, try to find the unsalted or the low-salt ones; all that salt will not be good for you in other respects, even if you are keeping your blood-sugar levels low!

Low-Carb Substitutes

There are many low-carb substitutes and the list is growing every day. As more and more research validates low-carb diet both for health and blood-sugar control, this field is going to explode. Already regular grocery stores carry low-carb bread and low-carb bars. In days to come this category of foods can only increase.

The best advice I can give you is to tell you to listen to Diana Ross's mom. Remember that classic line? "My momma told me—'You'd better shop around.'" Get on the

Internet and check out the sources of low-carb products, such as the Atkins Center, Keto products, Low-carb Nexus, and numerous others. You will find some taste great, some pretty lousy, and some mediocre. The good news is, these products are only going to get better and better.

The *low-carb muffins* are my favorites. These muffins taste as good as regular muffins, contain a fraction of the carbs, and are a great addition to a meal. They are filling and help you not to miss bread nearly so much. I love almost all of them: poppy-seed, blueberry, and orange-cranberry are special favorites. A meat dish, a salad, and one of these muffins makes a pretty great meal. You will get filled (depending on your size and the size of your meat and salad) and you will walk away from the table with your blood sugar barely affected. What a blessing! Make a new batch of muffins every week, and let them be a complement to your breakfasts, lunches, and suppers throughout the week.

There are all kinds of *low-carb bars*. To be honest, most of these do not compare with a Snickers bar or a Nestle's Crunch. Some are actually quite good, and others only fair. But they are often as low as two to four grams of net carbs per bar, which is next to nothing. When you are going to a restaurant where you know your friends are going to be ordering a dessert with coffee after the meal, bring one of these babies in your pocket or purse. Order your coffee and enjoy. They may not taste like french-silk pie, but they're not too bad, and you will be doing your body an enormous favor.

Low-carb pasta has a ways to go in the taste department, as I said earlier. It comes in handy at times, though, and is worth having around the house to satisfy those spaghetti cravings, or whatever other pasta dishes you feel you can't live without. Until they come up with a better-tasting pasta (and they surely will) I'd rather have my spaghetti sauce on a generous helping of spaghetti squash, which is amazingly good.

When you check out some of the companies that offer low-carb substitutes, you will be amazed at just what a variety they offer. You will find low-carb chips, bread, syrup, shakes, bars, hot and cold cereals, pancake mixes, hamburger buns, tortilla shells, barbecue sauce, puddings, and a lot more. And this is only going to get better and better, as research continues to demonstrate the value of low-carb eating.

One type of pasta that actually tastes great is made by the Dreamfields company. This pasta is made in such a way that most of the carbs simply do not digest but go through your system. It looks like regular pasta, tastes every bit as good, and yet is far more "pancreas friendly." Try it, and test your blood sugar about an hour after you eat. Most people will be amazed and thrilled to find you can have spaghetti again!

Experiment widely and you will come up with your own favorites. Some of the products taste great but are a bit pricey for most budgets, such as the low-carb ice cream (available in some supermarkets). By the way, don't be fooled by buying ice cream that merely says "no sugar added." There will still be plenty of carbs from the milk used. I found this out one time when I had a large bowl of this ice cream and was shocked to find that my blood sugars had gone to about 180 an hour later. The ultimate test of a food, as far as blood sugar is concerned, is the amount of total carbs minus the amount of fiber carbs. And be careful to note serving sizes. Sometimes foods list serving sizes unrealistically small, to give you the impression that you are not getting that much sugar or that many calories. To get an accurate count, you may need to double, triple, or quadruple the grams of carbs, depending on how much you eat!

Snacks

While snacks are not absolutely necessary, they provide an added boost of energy and sense of satisfaction in between your main meals. Those taking insulin usually don't want to go too long without eating, since they can run the risk of having a hypoglycemic episode. Likewise those who have developed insulin resistance, but whose pancreases are still fully functional, can stave off the fear of "blood-sugar jitters" by having a snack in between meals. (Although if you stay with a low-carb diet, this problem will take care of itself.)

At any rate most people like to have an occasional snack, and the trick is to be very much aware of the kinds of snacks that you can enjoy without driving your blood-sugar levels off the charts. Let me introduce to you the amazing Wasa cracker. (Actually, Wasa is simply the brand name, and you can find similar crackers with other names.)

A Wasa cracker is a flatbread cracker made of whole grains. Because it is so hard and flat it doesn't contain many carbs. Most have a carb content of seven grams with a fiber content of two grams, providing only five net grams of carbs for your pancreas to deal with. Of course you wouldn't want to eat these crackers by themselves. There are many low-carb choices to put on them: tuna salad, cream cheese, sliccd cheese, lunch meat, peanut butter (I told you I was a nut lover!), and ham would be good choices. One such cracker with a low-carb topping can be quite filling and easily last most people until their next meal.

Celery is extremely low in carbs. Smear some kind of low-carb product such as peanut butter or cream cheese and you have another tasty snack. A simple piece of cheese, a handful of nuts, a large piece of beef jerky, a pickle or a sliced cucumber, or a piece of low-carb bread with peanut butter and low-carb jelly can also tide you over nicely until dinnertime. Many times on trips I put peanut butter on a slice of low-carb bread, fold the bread in half, and put it in a plastic sandwich bag. I slip the bag in my sport-jacket pocket and know that I'm set for the day. The key is think these things through in advance. Don't wait until you get ravenous to try desperately to find something to eat. Too often you will compromise and end up eating something you shouldn't.

Using the Glucometer

I cannot overemphasize the importance of the glucometer in your early stages of rethinking your diet. Your glucometer will testify to the effectiveness of the low-carb diet. It will tell you what you can handle and what you can't. Learn to be comfortable with this invaluable aid.

I would encourage you to keep a record of your meals and how they register on the glucometer one to one and one half hours after you have finished eating. This will not only open your eyes, but it will give you a tremendous incentive to behave yourself, and receive the reward of a great blood-sugar reading. If you do splurge and eat too many foods you know you shouldn't, test yourself afterwards. The high blood-sugar reading will sicken your heart and give you a greater desire to follow the rules in the future.

You will learn what you can have and what you cannot. If you are truly diabetic, and your doctor will be able to tell you this, you will probably need to keep track of your blood-sugar levels daily for the rest of your life. If you are in a pre-diabetic state, you may get to the point where you can follow the low-carb diet and not need to check your levels so often.

Keep in mind that a person whose pancreas works well, and is not insulin-resistant, will have blood-sugar readings between 80 to 120. They will be at the low end of this when they first wake up and might reach the high end after a spaghetti dinner, with baked potato and French bread. If after such a meal, your blood sugar reaches 150 or more, you have blood-sugar problems and need to take the necessary steps to prevent full-blown diabetes. If your blood sugar rises over 200 at times, you should see a doctor, who will probably tell you that you are diabetic.

The wonderful thing about blood-sugar problems is that in most cases, if it is caught in the early stages, you can absolutely control your blood sugar with diet and moderate exercise. When I have a dinner of a steak, a salad with ranch dressing, and a low-carb muffin, there is no need for me to check my blood sugar. I know it will be fine. This is not necessarily true for the person with severe diabetes however; you check your blood-sugar levels as often as your doctor tells you! If I have my coffee at night with a low-carb syrup for sweetener and a low-carb bar with a few peanuts, checking my blood levels would be unnecessary. I haven't ingested enough carbs to make any real difference. I can go to sleep at ease, knowing that I am not going to awaken with any blood-sugar jitters.

The mighty little glucometer was a gift from God for me. It taught me, motivated me, and encouraged me. It brought me from a fear of the unknown to the confidence that I could, by the grace of God, win over this monster called diabetes.

One more word about these instruments. Don't pay any attention to those commercials that make you think it is terrible to stick your poor itty-bitty fingers with their terrible needles, attempting to scare you into spending more money on a fancier unit. In truth you will hardly feel the prick they make, and they almost never leave a mark or cause lasting soreness. A minute after taking your blood sugar, your finger will have forgotten its ordeal, but your mind will be better informed and your heart more strongly motivated, either by the pain of a bad reading or the pleasure of a good one.

Carb-Sparing

You would be amazed at just how many carbs you can spare yourself with just a little knowledge and a little willpower. Lets take a look at a typical McDonald's meal. You have just promised your kids that they could have

Happy Meals tonight. But what will you eat? The old, unconcerned, carb-ignorant you would have had something like your kids will have: a quarter-pounder, a large order of fries, a shake, and an apple pie for dessert. Such a meal has an enormous amount of carbs in it, more carbs than you should be eating in a day:

Item	Grams of Carbs
hamburger (actually the buns provide the carbs)	38
large order of fries	50
large Coke	60
apple pie	60
Total	**208**

If you are diabetic or insulin-resistant, you have just put your body under tremendous duress. You have dumped huge amounts of sugar into your bloodstream. If your pancreas still works, it will be pumping its guts out for the next couple of hours; if it doesn't, your blood sugar will rise dramatically.

Now let's look at a more sensible approach. Suppose you take the top bun off your hamburger. You have just reduced the carbs by about two thirds. Instead of ordering the large fries you order a vegetable salad with ranch dressing. Instead of a regular Coke you order a diet Coke (which has no carbs at all). And instead of the apple pie, you satisfy yourself with a low-carb bar you brought from home. (McDonald's won't mind. If they say anything, tell them I said it's okay.)

Look at the difference:

Item	Grams of Carbs
hamburger (with bottom bun only)	17
salad with dressing	8
diet Coke	0
low-carb bar	4
Total	**29**

What an incredible difference a few simple substitutions make! You will leave the table nearly as full, you will have enjoyed your meal and even had a "sweet" at its end, and yet you have just spared your body a major metabolic trauma. Do this once and that's good. Do this type of thing regularly and you could be on your way to a lifetime of freedom from blood-sugar problems. Of course you could have done better by doing away with the bun altogether, but eating the lower portion helps you to feel like you're still eating a hamburger, and can make your new lifestyle a little easier to take over the long haul.

Remember that you are not attempting to do away with carbs altogether. Such an approach would be unnecessary and unhealthy. You are simply needing to limit the carbs to a more natural level, and to make up for the fact that your body just doesn't process carbs the way it used to when you were 15.

For Travelers

For those who travel, continental breakfasts provided by most motels are a disaster. Almost everything they offer is pure carbs: bagels, doughnuts, cereal, and so on. When I arrive at a motel, I will go down to the breakfast the first day to see if there is anything worth eating. If not, I will either eat out or stay in my room and eat low-carb cereal I have brought with me. But often they do serve boiled eggs. Two of these, along with a low-carb muffin (which I am almost never without) make a fine breakfast. At my old weight of nearly 200 pounds this would not have filled me up, but at my new lifestyle weight of 165, I can do nicely with this breakfast. Besides I will have my low-carb 10:15 snack in a while, usually consisting of a Wasa cracker with sliced chicken and cheese. This tides me over until lunchtime.

Breakfasts at restaurants are easy: an omelet is perfect. It is tasty, high in protein, has almost no carbs to it, and is filling. Add a low-carb muffin (I sneak these in, in the pocket of my sport jacket), a cup of coffee, and you've got yourself a great breakfast. Life is good!

For example, consider the breakfasts that are served at IHOP, which are typical of American breakfast fare. IHOP serves its omelets with three pancakes. I eat one half pancake with my omelet. I ask for sugar free syrup, which tastes great and has no carbs. Again, the half pancake is not a serious challenge to my body, and it keeps me from feeling I can never eat a pancake again. It also goes great with the coffee! However I hasten to add that this is an exception, and not my usual practice when I am at home.

One basic rule at meals is not to have more than one high-carb item per meal. If you have some rice as a side dish, don't have beans as well. If you have a slice of bread, don't have pasta. And definitely don't have a sugary dessert. There really isn't much compromise you can allow yourself when it comes to pies, cakes, doughnuts, ice cream, and so forth. Go for the low-carb substitutes which can still please your sweet tooth without attacking your system. When it comes to regular desserts, just say no!

Nutritional Supplements

In theory, people who eat a healthy variety of foods should not need to take vitamin supplements. In practice this is almost never the case. Because a low-carb diet is going to limit your intake of fruits, which unquestionably are an excellent source of vitamins, you will need to take vitamin supplements. The truth is, if you do it right you will probably get as many or more vitamins than most Americans who eat a high-carb diet. You will be eating lots of salads, and if you make sure to include a great variety of veggies in those salads, along with spinach and other greens, you will almost certainly be ahead of the game.

That having been said, taking a vitamin is such a low-cost, low-effort procedure, there is no reason for you not to be taking advantage of the plethora of nutritional supplements available. I would recommend a multivitamin and mineral daily supplement, along with other supplements of your choice. There are lots of books and pamphlets available on vitamin supplements, and I am no expert, so I will not try to get into specifics, but please, please, at the very least go to Wal-Mart and get a daily vitamin and take it religiously. And eat lots of salads and veggies, along with berries, melons, and occasional tangerines. Don't turn the low-carb diet into a meat and cheese diet. (That's just stupid, if you'll pardon my bluntness.) Meat and cheese aren't nearly as bad as the "experts" have made them, but you cannot live on them alone. Most vegetables are low in carbs and high in vitamins—potatoes, corn, and carrots being the major exceptions. So indulge often in the low-carb veggies!

When it comes to tailoring an eating plan for the rest of your life, you are the ultimate authority. If you are fully diabetic you should certainly coordinate your efforts with a doctor. But by all means find a doctor who stresses diet and exercise along with medication, not one who will simply put you on insulin and say little about the factors you can control.

You cannot afford to neglect this business of diet. You can exercise three hours a day, but if you go on eating as you have before you are still likely to have problems. You must, absolutely must, find a way to radically reduce your intake of carbohydrates. And be sure to check out the companies that specialize in low-carb products. Get their catalogs and try all kinds of foods. You will be thrilled as you watch your blood-sugar levels begin to normalize. It feels good to win!

CHAPTER 9

The Second Front: Exercise

Somebody once wrote, "If the benefits of exercise were concentrated in a pill, everyone in America would be taking it." Exercise is one thing that the "experts" from all health branches and backgrounds agree upon. We should all be doing it.

As long as we only see exercise as a vague benefit that we *should* all be doing, and not as a specific, powerful tool in overcoming blood-sugar woes and staving off diabetes, we will probably not get all that serious. Exercise is so... sweaty! It is hard work, it is usually not all that fun, and to keep at it week in, week out, month in, month out, year in, year out, until we finally exit this life is quite an achievement.

You will never know just how far you can rise above your blood-sugar problems until you are making exercise an integral part of your daily routine. Those who say they don't have time to exercise are under a great delusion. If you knew how things truly are, you would say that you cannot afford not to exercise. Time spent in bringing our flabby bodies into a state of fitness is time well spent.

Knowledge Is Power

Information and motivation are tied together. The more good information you have, the more motivated you tend to be. The information is not hard to find. Study after study has indicated that exercise contains a plethora of benefits for nearly everyone. Your body was made to be used. The couch potato is living a lifestyle that contradicts the way he was made. Until the last hundred years, men and women have used walking as their primary means of transportation, have worked vigorously almost all of their lives. They had no televisions, no computers, and no video games to force them to sit for hours at a time, exercising only their fingers.

Remember this? "What you don't use, you lose." The "losing" process does not happen immediately, and this fact leads to an illusion. You can live without vigorous physical activity for decades and stay relatively healthy. For this reason, young people can laze around, eat poorly, sleep till noon (when they don't have school), and still have excellent blood-sugar response to the carbohydrates in their diet.

In the Bible we read about King David as an old man (he was in his late 60s and had lived a rough life) being cold all the time. They found a beautiful young lady to sleep with him to keep him warm. And in his condition sleep was all that went on. While we don't know his exact medical condition, it seems as though his metabolic system had slowed to a crawl. His circulation was so poor that his body was never warm enough. He had also lost his sexual desire to the degree that sleeping with a beautiful young woman never went beyond sleep.

This is an extreme example of what is gradually happening to all of us. We all joke about turning 40, and how the weight starts to come on after that. Well, it's no joke. It is certainly true. Most of us with kids have at least one child who eats like a pig and looks like a scarecrow. It seems they can eat mounds of doughnuts, huge platefuls of spaghetti, Big Macs galore, and down gallons of Coke without the slightest weight gain. The reason has to do with their metabolism. They are so metabolically wound up that they burn calories and process carbs with the greatest of ease.

It won't last forever. It is a sad fact of life that as we age, our metabolism and circulation gradually get slower and slower and slower. It is worse for some than for others, but all will experience this to one degree or another. Along with a decreased metabolism, blood pressure tends to rise, arteries tend to clog, and our mechanisms for processing glucose become more and more inefficient. This is why 50- and 60-year-olds have lots more heart attacks and diabetes than 18- and 20-year-olds.

While we aren't going to be able to overcome aging, there are some steps we can take to stave off some of its most destructive effects. Exercise is one of the most beneficial of those steps. When you raise your normal heartbeat to a significant degree, you force your metabolism to speed up, as though you were years younger. Your circulation increases dramatically, your blood flows freely, your heart is strengthened, and your arteries and veins receive a cleansing. Obviously we can't exercise all day long, nor would it be good for us. It is only necessary for us to exercise a relatively brief portion of our day (30 minutes to an hour) in order for us to reap incredible benefits.

Exercise and Blood Sugar

Study after study continually demonstrates the value of exercise as it relates to both heart health and improved blood-sugar efficiency. At a symposium on diabetes at Boston University Medical Center, Dr. Neil Ruderman noted, "Exercise can improve insulin action—helping control or even prevent type 2 diabetes—and also may help lower blood pressure and lipid abnormalities that contribute to heart disease." Another speaker at the symposium, Dr. Ralph Paffenberger of Stanford University School of Medicine, stated, "The risk of type 2 diabetes is reduced by 25% and of heart disease by 50% among people who are moderately vigorously active."

Lifestyle or Medication?

Thousands of adults across the country at high risk for type 2 diabetes joined a research study called the Diabetes Prevention Program (DPP). Everyone in the study had impaired glucose tolerance (in other words, their bodies didn't handle sugar very well) and was overweight. They divided volunteers into the following groups: 1) lifestyle change (exercise, diet, and weight control), 2) taking the oral diabetes drug metformin (Glucophage) twice a day, or 3) receiving a placebo. As expected, both the lifestyle change group and the metformin group achieved improvements in their blood-sugar levels and ability to tolerate glucose, but they didn't realize just how much more effective the lifestyle change would be!

These people were not diabetics, but were one step away from becoming diabetics. Those who took the metformin cut the incidence of new cases of diabetes by 31 percent—but those who adopted only the lifestyle changes cut their incidence of diabetes by a whopping 58 percent! "What floored us was how quickly diet and exercise made a big impact in reversing the slide into diabetes," reported Mary Hoskin, the coordinator of the clinical trial in Arizona. "In just 3 years, diet and exercise resulting in a modest weight loss of, say, 10 or 15 pounds made such a big difference in health."[7]

Thus, one fourth of all type 2 diabetics don't have to be diabetics at all—if they would only exercise. This does not include dealing with the other two disciplines: proper weight and diet. If just exercise alone can cut your chances of diabetes by one fourth, how much better will it be for those who not only exercise but also maintain the proper weight and eat a healthy, low-carb diet?

Doctor and author Joseph Mercola has himself struggled with diabetes. He jogs 20 miles each week and notes, "When I reduce my miles to 5 or less (per week), my blood sugar gradually rises to the diabetic range. One does not have to run 20 miles per week, but most diabetics will benefit from forty minutes to one hour of intense exercise at least five times per week, and more if their blood-sugar is out of control."[6] The beauty of what Dr. Mercola discovered is that he has a lot to say about his blood-sugar levels. Stay at the 20 miles per week and everything is fine. Drop down to just a few miles and he is a diabetic. He determines whether he is a diabetic or not. What a far cry from the standard "take a pill and do what you like" approach of so many type 2 diabetics!

Dr. Michael D. Brown and his colleagues at the University of Pittsburgh enrolled 12 overweight African–American women in a seven-day exercise program. Their daily routine consisted of a 10-minute warm-up (walking and stretching) followed by 30 minutes of aerobic exercise (treadmill, brisk walking, or cycling), 5 minutes of rest, and then 20 additional minutes of aerobic exercise. After only a week, they found the women's insulin sensitivity had improved by 58 percent! This is incredible. Lack of insulin sensitivity is what makes type 2 diabetics. A 58 percent gain in insulin sensitivity can make the difference between blood-sugar levels that rise to 150 after a meal and those that stay in the safe 120 range. Again, if you can see these kinds of gains by only adding exercise to your life, how much more can you expect if you add exercise, plus diet, plus the proper weight!

I recall watching a piece on *Prime Time Live* about diabetes in American Indians quite a few years ago. Diabetes hits American Indians worse than any other race or culture. This program focused upon one tribe where they were coming down with diabetes in tremendous numbers. Many of the members of this tribe decided to take up jogging, some as a preventative measure and others as a means to control the diabetes they already had. As they jogged, their blood sugars came under control. One man told how he had had blood-sugar levels five times the norm (500 mg/dl) and after getting seriously into jogging he was now in the normal range. When I first suspected I either had diabetes or something that could easily turn into it, I immediately thought of that Indian man, and I determined that exercise was going to be a part of my life from here on!

Types of Exercise

There are basically two types of exercise: aerobic and resistance. In simple terms, aerobic exercise is where you get your heart rate up and keep it up for a relatively lengthy period of time. Aerobic exercises would include brisk walking, jogging, swimming, rowing, cycling, etc. When you practice this kind of endurance exercise, all sorts of things change in your body. Your face may get red, your heart rate increases, you usually begin to sweat, your blood thins out and circulates much more freely, and you start huffing and puffing (especially if you're not in shape). *You were made to do this frequently!* For most of recorded history, men and women worked hard and walked briskly for many miles each week. What is most unnatural is to wake up, gorge down two jelly doughnuts with a cup of coffee, go to work and sit at a desk for eight hours, come home, eat half a pizza with a large Coke, slump onto a couch and watch TV for four hours, and then go to bed.

While you may not be able to do anything about your desk job, you can overcome the negative effects of eight hours of sitting with 40 minutes of brisk aerobic exercise five to six days each week. If you don't yet have diabetes this can delay its onset for 20 years, 30 years, or even a lifetime. If you do have it, aerobic exercise can be of tremendous value in keeping your blood sugars under control, and immunizing yourself from all the deleterious effects that normally come with diabetes. And while you are at it, you just might be saving yourself from a heart attack as well!

The benefits of aerobic exercise are so bountiful that a person would be foolish not to do it, even if he had no blood-sugar problems at all. If you do have blood-sugar issues, it is an absolute must for you. Your fasting blood-sugar level will come down, your insulin resistance will significantly decrease, and your body will become efficient once again at processing carbs and glucose. You won't get your teenage body back (sorry to say!) but you will get the next best thing: You will regain much of your body's metabolic efficiency. This is no license for you to go to your nearest pizza parlor and pig out, however. The key to overcoming diabetes is not diet *or* exercise; it is diet *plus* exercise (plus weight maintenance).

The other type of exercise is known by various names: anaerobic, resistance training, and so forth. It involves muscle toning. The goal here is not to huff and puff for half an hour, but rather to turn flab into muscle through repetitive sets of muscle flexes. Weight lifting, push-ups, and sit-ups would all be examples of resistance training. At one time most of the "experts" were giving little heed to resistance training as a benefit to people with blood-sugar concerns. That has changed.

Today, more and more evidence has come in that resistance training is as good for the diabetic as aerobic exercise is. For one thing, researchers have discovered that muscle is far more efficient at processing glucose than fat. The person with rolls of fat around his middle and on his thighs is going to start out with two strikes against him. Even if he loses no weight, if he can simply turn much of that fat into muscle, he will see better blood-sugar levels. It is no marvel that overweight people have such excellent chances to become diabetics. They usually have little muscle tone, they are carrying too many pounds, and they are almost always eating poorly and too much. They are a diabetic time bomb waiting to explode!

To beat diabetes you must take advantage of every weapon available. Don't just pick up your rifle and leave the hand grenades on the ground. Don't just call for the artillery and ignore the air force. (I bet you can tell I like military history, can't you?) In the context of exercise you cannot focus only upon aerobic exercise and neglect resistance training. You must do both.

Aerobic Exercise

There are differences of opinion as to how much time you should spend in aerobic exercise in order for it to do you the most good. There are also differing ideas as to just how tough such exercise must be. Some have suggested that even a light walk for 20 minutes, three times a week, will provide major benefits. Others have not been so generous, and insisted that it should be much more vigorous exercise, and should be at least five days a week, 45 minutes a day.

Keep in mind that you are fighting a vicious foe. Diabetes wants to take your limbs, your ability to walk, your joy, your peace, and eventually your life. You cannot approach the battle lightly. For you to do a mild little 15-minute walk a couple of times a week is not going to make much difference. You are going to have to get serious about this business of exercise.

The other side of the coin is that you don't have to be an Olympic athlete to win this battle, either. One of the keys is to stay at whatever aerobic exercise you choose for at least 40 minutes each time you do it. Of course there may be days when you have to shorten it to 30 for time's sake, but let that be the exception and not the rule! Four days each week is probably the minimum you should exercise. Five days a week and 40 minutes each day will come out to three hours and 20 minutes a week. Each week contains 168 hours, so we're not talking about something impossible here. Anyone who is so busy that they cannot designate a little over three hours a week for the sake of their health is too busy!

I have mentioned it already, but I must say it again. As far as I'm concerned the treadmill is the ideal exercise machine. It can be set up in front of a TV, it can be programmed to run at the speed you decide is ideal for you, and you will either keep up with that speed or be thrown off the machine. Because it is right there in your home, weather will not affect you, nor will it take excess time to get to your starting point, as it does when you have to drive to a fitness club.

But that's just me. You may find the treadmill a drag and opt for a cross-country skiing machine, or a stationary bicycle. Just make sure you get moving fast enough to break a sweat, and get that heart pumping. Don't go so fast that you wear yourself out, though. Firstly that's not good for you, and secondly you would never be able to keep up that kind of regimen for a lifetime. Work at a rate of exercise that is a challenge, but not a terror! Find something you can live with, and then live with it.

The Promise of Mornings

Allow me to say something about mornings. Mornings are wonderful. There is no time of day quite so full of promise or so beautiful as the mornings. Tasks that are done in the morning are tasks that always get done. You say you're not a morning person? Let the morning work for you.

Why am I going on so about mornings? Because I have seen over and over again that the best time to exercise is in the morning. Whenever I put off my exercise till the afternoon or evening, I find that the day has slipped away and I haven't exercised. I have seen this so many times, I have determined that whatever else I do or don't do in the morning, I will exercise. That way, regardless of how busy my day becomes later, the exercise will already have been safely completed.

There is another reason to exercise in the morning— a metabolic one. Your metabolism is always running at its slowest in the mornings. You have just been sleeping for seven or eight hours. Your entire body has been in the sleep mode. Your heart has been slowed way down, your circulation is sluggish, and your entire physical system is in need of a wake-up call. This tragedy is often compounded when diabetics or pre-diabetics eat a carb-laden breakfast. They stuff themselves with pancakes drenched with sugary syrup, or they down two or three bowls of cereal loaded with carbs, or eat several large biscuits with gravy.

These high-carb meals would be a challenge to your body at any time, but how much more so when you have just been up a little while! The key to getting off to a great day of low blood-sugar levels is to eat a low-carb breakfast and then spend about 40 to 45 minutes of aerobic exercise. By the way, this is also true of naps. One of the highest blood-sugar levels I ever recorded was after I had taken a good, long Sunday afternoon nap. I woke up and had a bowl of cereal. (I was still experimenting and learning in those days—I would not do such a thing today.) My blood-sugar level rose to over 200 and stayed high for several hours. It was a depressing situation, but I learned that cereal, which was one of the last high-carb foods I (reluctantly) gave up, would have to go. After a love affair of nearly 50 years, I finally received the grace to say, "Hasta la vista, baby!" My blood-sugar levels have been better ever since. (They are starting to make low-carb cereals that aren't too bad.)

Resistance Exercise

Because resistance exercise tones your body and turns fat into muscle, it is a useful tool. The goal is not to look like Arnold Schwarzenegger! You don't have to become a massive hulk to do yourself some good. The beauty of resistance exercise is that it can be worked into your schedule at almost any time, and it doesn't require a whole lot of it to do you good.

You will gain the most benefit by developing your larger muscles. Specifically these are the chest, thighs, and shoulders. My muscles of choice are the chest muscles. These muscles seem to grow and develop faster than all other muscles and respond beautifully to even fairly small sets of repetitions. To develop the chest muscle, let me recommend the common push-up. The beauty of the push-up is that it requires no special equipment other than a floor, which is almost always available. I have found that four or five sets of push-ups, done three times a week, are enough to provide wonderful results both in size and strength of the chest muscles.

When I began to do push-ups I could barely do ten or twelve. As I began a thrice weekly regimen, I steadily gained in strength and size. Before long I was doing 20 at a time, then 25. Soon I could do 40 on a good day. I usually start out with a lower amount on my first rep, and then increase with each set I do. I try to do several sets of push-ups in the morning, such as when I first get up, before I do the treadmill, and after the treadmill. Sometimes I do a set or two at work. Because 30 or 40 push-ups can be done in about a minute, they require a minimal time factor and do you a major benefit. Four or five sets a day three times a week is enough to keep your muscles toned and make a difference in your blood-sugar readings. While resistance training is not the most potent weapon in the bag, it is a significant one, and it is something that we all can find time to do, with a little bit of discipline. We are talking about between 15 minutes to 40 minutes a week here, with the sets worked in between other activities. You can do this!

"Weight Transfer"

Keep in mind that when you develop muscles in one part of your body, your body is going to transfer weight from other parts to sustain your new muscles. Thus, if you stay at the same weight, but increase your chest muscles, chances are your waistline will decrease at least a little. Every little bit you can take off your waist is vitally important. Researchers have found a direct correspondence between the size of the belly and the incidence of diabetes. People who store their fat on their thighs are far less likely to develop diabetes as people who store their weight on their stomach. In other words, for blood-sugar efficiency, lose that gut!

Sit-ups are good for turning stomach fat into muscles but are one of my least favorite exercises. I have found that by staying at the proper weight and developing my chest muscles, I keep my stomach at a reasonable size. My waist is 34 inches, which is two inches more than my high school years. I tend to store my weight in my stomach, so this is not too bad for me. If I weighed 240 pounds, I would probably still have skinny arms and legs, and a massive belly. Today, my stomach still has a slight bulge, but if I dropped much more weight, I would look like I had come out of a concentration camp in all the other parts of my body.

Leg lifts are the preferred exercise for firming up thigh muscles. If you prefer to use weights, the bench press is pretty much the equivalent of the push-up. Curls with barbells can build up your biceps. Lifting a bar from the shoulders to the head will build up your shoulder muscles. I will not presume to tell you what type of resistance program to employ, but I do encourage you to do something. You were not created to be flabby! Fat, flabby people with almost no muscle tone will sooner or later pay the consequences for their self-indulgence. Our bodies were meant to be pushed and challenged, both in terms of endurance (aerobic exercises) and strength (anaerobic exercises).

Can women benefit from resistance training? Absolutely! Women are never going to look like Mr. Schwarzenegger (praise the Lord!) because their muscles don't bulk up the way men's muscles do. This is the way your Creator made you. You don't have a lot of choice in this. But women can firm up their flab through resistance training and make their bodies far more efficient in sugar processing capability.

Don't strain yourself! As you do your reps, don't carry them out until you can do no more. Always stop a little short of your max. You won't do yourself any favor by pulling a muscle and making it impossible for you to exercise for the next two weeks. Work your body hard, but don't abuse it.

Motivation

You are going to be doing this for the rest of your life. For the sake of your loved ones who will be blessed by you living a long life, and for the sake of all the other people your long life will touch, on the practical side you will need to take some steps to ensure that you don't bog down in the process. A few people on this planet are self-motivated to the extreme and rarely need any help to do the things they should. For all the rest of us, we need some encouragement and a little wisdom to help us stay the course.

Exercise is not inherently fun. Once I had a neighbor describing his hobby of metal-detecting to me. He made the statement, "Yeah, it's kind of fun for me, sort of like you are with jogging." (At that time I was jogging outdoors regularly.) I couldn't let that one pass. I told him, "Jogging's no fun for me. I don't take any pleasure in it." He asked, "Then why do you do it?" Of course I told him I did it for health reasons.

Exercise, by definition, does not rank up there with eating and sex. Therefore, any pleasure you can work into it is well worth it, as we tend to stay with those things we enjoy and give up on those things we don't. There are several ways to do this. My preferred way, as I have already mentioned, is to hook up headphones to my sound system and listen to history documentaries and historical movies on TV as I exercise. Some people might think us strange to have a treadmill in our living room, but my health is well worth the price of having a few people think I'm a little strange.

Other motivational steps could include listening to tapes or CDs of your favorite preacher or books, listening to your favorite type of music, walking outdoors with a friend, or varying the types of exercise you do to keep things fresh. You might do cycling one month, treadmill the next, outdoor walks the next, and so forth.

If you get so busy you don't get a chance to exercise on a day you planned to, make sure to get back to your routine the next day. One of the great killers of exercise plans is the law of inertia. Once you have gone a couple of weeks without exercise, the law of inertia kicks in, and it will require a major effort to begin anew. For this reason you cannot let one missed day turn into a week of missed days.

As one day follows another, and the months go by, your exercise will become an integral part of your life. As your muscles and your cardiovascular system respond to the new demands you place on them, you will find the exercises aren't nearly the pain that they were at first. (No, they probably will never reach the "whoopee" category, but they will not seem like too much of a burden.) In truth your exercise program is doing for you what normal life did for your ancestors. By keeping your body active you will slow down the degeneration of your metabolism and even the aging process. You will be more likely to have normal blood pressure and much less likely to have a stroke. Your body's cells will handle blood sugar more efficiently, and your daily blood-sugar levels will move toward normal. And the decades of health you will likely receive will more than compensate for the 40 minutes you spend in daily exercise.

CHAPTER 10

The Third Front: Weight

Every war has certain fronts that are tougher and nastier than the others. Weight is not one of them! The idea that losing weight or maintaining weight is some undefeatable monster is a falsehood. Actually, losing weight is pretty much a given to overweight people who will fight diligently on the first two fronts: diet and exercise.

If you consistently eat a low-carb diet and exercise 40 minutes a day, six days a week, you will have a hard time staying overweight. It's just that simple! Now there are some weight-loss techniques that I will share with you in this chapter, but these are not the keys to victory. The keys are in the previous two chapters. Let me repeat it: It will be extremely difficult for you to stay overweight if you eat right and exercise. It can be done, but you will have to work at it.

Why Diets Don't Work

It is a fact of life that diets do not work for the vast majority of people who employ them. Americans have had diets of every possible type thrust at them over the years. Some diets have been fairly sound; others extremely flaky. But the one thing that they have in common is that people nearly always fail to meet their goal or attain that goal for any reasonable length of time. What to do then? Some give up and indulge (usually feeling guilty and not very good about themselves), while others search for a new diet, a new method, a new health and fitness guru who can lead them into the promised land of slimness and fitness.

I am no health guru. I'm not a health "nut." I am a simple preacher who, out of necessity, searched for and discovered a few of the basic keys to health that really work in the physical realm. It all has to do with natural versus unnatural. Banana splits and rolls of flab around your waist are not natural. Salads, meats, nuts, and cheese are. Sitting at a computer chair for eight hours at work, and then on a couch for six more hours at home, is not natural. Getting your body moving, your heart pumping, and your sweat glands sweating is.

When it comes to weight loss, the reason for the extreme failure rate of diets is that they are just that— they are diets. And in our popular culture a diet is not a style of eating, but rather a prescribed way of eating used as a tool to arrive at a definite goal. Thus if you are on the "bananas and peanut butter diet" you will eat nothing but bananas and peanut butter for the next X number of months until you reach your ideal weight of 130 or 165 or whatever. You see the bananas and the peanut butter as a tool, the way a mechanic sees his wrench or a carpenter his circular saw. Tools are made to be used for specific purposes and laid down.

So it is with your "diet." You will live on bananas and peanut butter only until you "get there," and then you will drop it like a hot (high-carb) potato! After all, you would be crazy to try and live on bananas and peanut butter for the next several decades.

This is even true with the fancy dinners that certain weight-loss programs offer. The dinners are tasty, fairly nutritious...and cost a fortune. You don't have any intentions of eating these dinners for the rest of your life. They will be helpful in losing some pounds, but after that you will go back to regular foods—and gain the weight right back!

Herein lies the problem, as well as the implied answer. In order to lose weight and maintain that weight loss, you will have to find a "diet" that you can live with—a diet in the truly best sense of the word. As one who is either diabetic or pre-diabetic you have a built-in incentive that other people do not have. If you have any idea of just how bad diabetes is, and what it can cost you, you will have a motivation far stronger than others to move to a diet more conducive to weight loss (and blood-sugar control) and stay with it.

In order for you to be able to live with a diet for the next several decades, your diet will need to meet the following conditions:

1. It should not be drab or tasteless.
2. It should consist of foods that are not overexpensive. (Who could afford a caviar diet?)
3. It should not leave you constantly hungry.
4. It should not require extraordinary time to produce the meals.
5. It should include enough variation so as not to be boring.
6. It should not tax your pancreas.
7. It should include an ample supply of vitamins and minerals.

The No-Diet Diet

The low-carb diet fills every one of the above needs. But the amazing thing about it is that it really isn't a diet at all in the way most people think of diets. For example, when eating low-carb meals you are not required to think much about portions or calories. The reason for this is twofold. First, a low-carb diet results in far less insulin coursing through your veins, which means you end up burning fat more efficiently. You can actually ingest more calories and still lose weight. Secondly, many of the low-carb foods you will eat are not calorie-dense. Your stomach will get filled before you can gorge on enough calories to add on the pounds.

This points to a basic truth. Oftentimes, people are not

overweight because they eat too much, but because they eat too much of the wrong foods. Having your stomach filled after a meal is not a problem. Having your stomach filled with high-calorie foods after a meal most certainly is.

Consider the lowly salad. A stomach full of salad is probably not going to cause you to gain any weight at all. A stomach full of coconut cream pie will, as will a stomach full of jelly doughnuts, lasagna, or cherry cheesecake.

Now, we are not going to live on all salads, but if you eat a fairly large salad at dinner (with a lower calorie dressing), and then a reasonable portion of meat and a vegetable such as broccoli or cauliflower, you have just saved yourself a weight gain. Meat is not an especially low-calorie food, yet meat helps you lose weight because most of us find it difficult to "pig out" on meat. Now, we *do* pig out on meat-and-pasta dishes such as lasagna, spaghetti, or beef stroganoff, but to many people, a piece of meat by itself is not nearly the temptation that a plate of lasagna is.

It is possible to gain weight or to stay overweight on a low-carb diet, but it is not at all likely. As long as you stay with low-carb foods, you have an excellent chance that weight control will hardly be an issue. I am a perfect example of this. For several years my weight hovered in the high 180s and low 190s. My shirts were all tight on me, and my belly was the recipient of most of my extra weight (the very worst place for weight to accumulate for people with blood-sugar problems). After I set a few guidelines for losing weight and began to apply them conscientiously, the weight began to come off. By keeping to the rules of no second helpings, no eating between meals, low-cal salad dressings, and so forth, I was able to get to my target weight and stay there.

But once my blood-sugar problems motivated me to go to a low-carb diet, I found I could throw most of the rules out the window. I could eat between meals, I could eat second helpings, and I could enjoy high-fat salad dressings and still not gain weight. As a matter of fact, at first I had to hustle just to keep from losing too much weight and looking as skinny as a rail. After I discovered more low-carb choices of foods to eat and snack on, I was finally able to get up to 165 and stay there. I had dropped as low as 154 and looked way too thin.

So, for many of you, a low-carb diet may well be the only weight control measure you need. But for the sake of those who need a little extra help, I will go into a few basic principles of weight control.

Weight-Control Principle #1: Moderation

The Bible speaks of a virtue called moderation, which means "the quality of restraint; the avoidance of extremes." (Christian readers will recall that a moderate, self-controlled life is an extremely important aspect of basic Christianity.)

When it comes to eating, moderation means you don't eat until you are absolutely stuffed. You don't eat as much as your body would desire. You eat moderately. For someone who has spent a lifetime force-feeding himself, this seems like sheer agony. It feels almost criminal to leave the table without feeling stuffed. Let me give you a very profound bit of advice: Get used to it!

Weight-Control Principle #2: Slavery

Slavery means having no control. Slaves had no control over their lives. They worked at jobs decided for them by their masters, they lived where their masters told them to live, they ate the food provided by their masters, and they did whatever their masters told them to do. Their list of choices in life was almost nil. It was either obey or suffer severe punishment.

In the Bible, Jesus tells us wrongdoing has a similar effect. We find ourselves doing things we don't want to do, saying things we don't want to say, and living lives that fill us with guilt and regret. In the area of overeating, this is especially difficult. The alcoholic can at least swear off all forms of alcohol and remove himself from his nemesis. The drug addict can start hanging around a new crowd that doesn't do drugs and remove much of the temptation. But the foodaholic is still going to have to eat. Every meal, indeed every time he opens his mouth he is at risk of another binge.

Now, hear me out because I'm speaking from my own experience. The good news is, Jesus is in the deliverance business. He has come as a Savior—and that presupposes a condition of slavery and desperate need. He is the Answer to food slavery. (See appendix A for more on this.)

Weight-Control Principle #3: Accountability

Just as the glucometer is a powerful tool for evaluating your metabolic progress overall, the scale will be of immeasurable help in evaluating your success or failure in weight control. You should not get obsessed with your weight, but you should, in a reasonable fashion, keep tabs on it. Purchase a high-quality scale so that you won't be concerned with false reading. Weigh yourself at the same time every day. In the morning, before you eat or drink, is probably the best choice. That way you will get a more consistent picture of your progress.

Don't rush the weight loss. If you eat a low-carb diet, and eat reasonable portions, excess weight doesn't stand a chance of hanging around. You won't drop 50 pounds in a few weeks, but so what? You didn't gain all that weight in a few weeks, and it is silly to think you should lose it that way. People who lose weight too fast are excellent candidates for gaining it all back—with interest! You are not on a diet! You are on a lifestyle change. Don't skip meals, don't starve yourself, and enjoy your meals! Have a low-carb treat from time to time. Indulge in low-carb desserts occasionally. But keep the goal in mind.

When you get to your desired weight you cannot simply put the scale in the closet and eat as you will. Continue to weigh yourself, not necessarily every day, but every few days at least. When I first went on my low-carb diet I lost more weight than I needed to or wanted to, due to my limited repertoire of low-carb foods and desserts. As my repertoire increased I began moving toward my desired weight of 165. I have now been there for some time, and I find that if I totally ignore my dietary habits I tend to start to encroach upon the 170s. When the scale registers me at 167 or 168 I simply cut back a little. I don't starve myself, but I have lighter lunches and smaller snacks. Before long I drop down to where I want to be. It is not a major effort, but it does require vigilance.

Like the glucometer your scale provides two indispensable factors: evaluation and motivation. Your scale is not your enemy; it is your friend. Learn to see it that way.

Some Basic Rules for Losing Weight

I really don't much like "rules." They seem so confining. But the truth is, most of our success in life comes through following certain rules. (You can call them guidelines, principles, helps, or whatever else you want, if it makes you feel better!)

When it comes to weight loss, one thing is for certain. If you have a need to lose weight, you have been doing something wrong in the past. If you were doing everything right, you wouldn't need to be reading this chapter! And if you keep on doing what you have been doing, you will keep on being overweight and have excellent chances of becoming more overweight than ever before. Thus, some changes are going to have to occur. Here is a list of a few suggested changes that can make a big difference in your waistline—and in your facial expression when you step off the scale.

Rule #1: No Second Helpings

Most of the time we mean well. We take a reasonable portion of the various foods available. After all, we would look like too much of a glutton if we loaded our plate to its capacity—until the gravy spills over on one side and the beans on the other. Somehow we find that after we have finished our plate we are still just a wee bit hungry. Maybe a little extra meat, a few more potatoes, one more roll. After the second go-around, we might just snack on a few pretzels on our way from the table. Before we know it, we have consumed twice as much as was originally on our plate.

To lose weight and keep it off, one of the most powerful decisions you can make is *no second helpings*. You will place a reasonable amount of food on your plate, and when that runs out, you will shut down your stomach until the next meal. Not only will this keep you from all kinds of unwanted calories, but it will ensure you don't go into a cycle of skimping on dinner and then getting so hungry you find yourself inexorably drawn to the snack cabinet a couple of hours later. As you load your plate, ask yourself, Is this a responsible and reasonable meal? Knowing that the portions you take are all you're going to get will cause you to be a little more careful in taking slightly more than you might otherwise have done, but in the end you will come out way ahead.

Rule #2: Either No Snacks or Planned Snacks

Other than second helpings, the next greatest adversary of weight control is the in-between meal snack. Typically our breakfast and lunch are separated by about five hours, and our lunch and dinner by around five and one half hours. For many that is a long, long time to go without food. This is especially true for people eating foods with a high-carb content. Carbohydrates make us feel great when we are hungry, as they quickly raise our blood-sugar and energy levels. The problem is they are very much like kindling. They burn fast and they burn out fast. Before long their carbs have all been turned to sugar, our bodies have responded by producing lots and lots of insulin, and there are no more carbs to deal with. The excess insulin then drives our blood sugar much too low, and we get that jittery, nervous, "gotta get something to eat" feeling. Too often we find ourselves headed right back to the high-carb foods, and the cycle repeats itself.

When you eat a low-carb diet, you will not experience those drastic highs and lows and will find that you don't have such a desire to snack as before. But people being people, most of us still appreciate a little snack from time to time.

The Unplanned Snack

An occasional snack is not a problem as long as it is low-carb and planned. The enemy of weight loss is the unplanned snack. You find yourself hungry and you grab whatever is handy. Your friend offers you a bag of potato chips, and before you know it you have eaten half the bag. Bad, bad, bad! Chips and pretzels are the worst kind of snacks. They have far too much salt, almost no nutrition, and lots of calories. You'd be about as well-off if you ate cardboard. So if you decide you want to or need to snack, plan for it!

Plan a low-carb snack that will not drive your blood sugar into the stratosphere and will not be overloaded with calories. A rolled up ham slice and a piece of cheese, cream cheese on a Wasa cracker, celery with peanut butter are examples of low-carb snacks that are not going to have a significant effect upon your blood sugar. Half of a cucumber in slices is an excellent choice as cucumbers have so few carbs it's not worth mentioning. A handful of nuts would also be good. Check a food chart that displays the carb content for most foods, and you can make your own informed choices.

The diabetic whose pancreas no longer produces insulin (if this is your case your doctor will have you taking insulin shots) has slightly different needs concerning snacks. If you are in this category, you need to coordinate your snack regimen with your doctor, and to keep a close eye on your blood-sugar levels at different times throughout the day.

Rule #3: Substitute

This is a relatively pain-free means of reducing your total calories. You simply look for ways to substitute low-calorie foods and condiments for the high-calorie ones. Start out with sodas. Of course people with blood-sugar problems should never drink regular sodas anyway. The diet sodas have no calories, and even better, they have no carbohydrates. They are not going to be affecting your blood sugar, and at the same time they are going to be a calorie-free drink that tastes pretty good. Yes, I know they take a little getting used to, but they are not bad with those foods that seem to be incomplete without soda. I would not drink them too frequently, however, as NutraSweet, which is the primary sweetener in most diet sodas, can cause problems for some when taken in large quantities.

Salad dressings can be real killers in the calorie department. Often a couple of tablespoons of salad dressing will be more calories than all of your salad. They can take what appears to be a healthy, low-calorie food, and turn it into a sugary, calorie-laden food. Go for the low-carb and low-calorie salad dressings.

Of course, if you stay with a solid low-carb dietary plan, most of the substitutions will be unnecessary. I enjoy the high-fat salad dressings these days (but make sure they are low sugar), as weight has not been a problem for me in a long while. But in the beginning you may find it helpful to use some of the low-fat items to help in shedding those first pounds.

Keep in mind that many of these low-calorie items are labeled low-fat. The fat is not really your enemy; it just happens that low-fat foods are usually lower in calories. But don't fall into the "everything's got to be low-fat" mentality. As far as your health goes, it is the chips, the breads, the pasta, and the cakes and pies that are doing you in, not the fat. Nuts, which are high in fat, are wonderfully nutritious and heart-healthy. You may need to lay low on them at first until your weight gets under control, but don't give up on them. They are a gift from God! Two hundred calories' worth of nuts is infinitely better for you than 150 calories' worth of salted snack crackers made of refined flour and filled with blood-sugar-raising carbs.

Rule #4: Check the Calories

When it comes to weight control, many people are dying of ignorance. They are eating indiscriminately, never considering the source of their extra girth. Often it's not so much a matter of cutting down on food, but rather eating those foods which are not laden with the potential to puff you up like a balloon. For this reason you are going to have to become a label reader. Check out how many calories make up portions of your favorite foods. As you shop, compare brands and different kinds of foods, and make wise choices. There are Splenda-sweetened ice-cream bars that are as low as 35 calories and have about six net carbs. Don't just throw things into your shopping cart indiscriminately. If you make wise decisions at the grocery store you won't need to count calories at each meal.

Lifestyle, Lifestyle, Lifestyle

Let me close by reminding you once again that you are not going "on a diet." You are changing your eating and living habits for the rest of your life. Once you get close to your target weight, start buying yourself some new clothes. Throw out the old stuff; you'll never need it again. Your new, slimmer body will not only look better (which should be the least of your reasons for the change), but it will serve you better.

Most likely you will have added several years to your life. In some cases people will add several decades. These can be wonderful years to love your family and serve your God.

CHAPTER 11

Does Anyone Have a Question?

One of the disadvantages of reading a book on health as opposed to attending a live seminar is that you don't get to ask any of the many questions that come to mind. Drawing on the material in the previous chapters, I have tried to anticipate some of the questions that may be rising in your mind and answer them concisely.

1. Is this diet safe?

This is a fair question. After all, it's not much help if you bring your blood sugar under control and then end up dying of a heart attack and clogged arteries. Here are the two biggest concerns about a low-carb diet:

1. Does it raise your cholesterol levels and lead to heart problems?

2. Won't you suffer nutritionally?

The first question has been thoroughly answered by many studies that have been done over the last decade. Study after study reveals that people who maintain a strict low-carb diet do not raise their total cholesterol. As a matter of fact their total cholesterol almost always decreases. Tremendous results have been shown in triglyceride levels as well. This has been a most perplexing issue for the low-fat pushing medical "experts" who have loudly insisted that such a diet is "absolutely crazy." To their chagrin, all the major indicators of health seem to improve when people begin to eat the low-carb way.

Keep these two things in mind. While it is true you will be eating more protein and ingesting greater amounts of cholesterol, it does not necessarily follow that you will be loading your body with that cholesterol. You will be getting more fat by eating a little more meat than you perhaps used to, but you will be getting far less fat from the sweets that used to be such a big part of your diet. The simple truth is this: America's heart problems do not come from her consumption of meat. Whole societies have eaten far more meat than we do and suffered almost no heart disease. Our problem has to do with the sweet rolls, pasta, doughnuts, cakes, pies, french fries, white bread, bagels, and all the other mega-carb foods that we eat, along with our meat. By these we turn our bodies into cholesterol-collecting machines, and the meat that we eat does indeed become problematic. You can eat meats and salads all your life and keep your cholesterol and triglycerides low. It is the eating of meat along with large doses of carbs that drives your cholesterol up and makes you a walking candidate for a heart attack.

As for nutritional needs, a low-carb diet could be a problem nutritionally, but it certainly doesn't have to be. If your idea of low-carbing it means huge steaks at every meal, along with cheese and eggs, and few or no vegetables, you *will* suffer nutritionally. Our loving Creator has given us the gift of vegetables, which are loaded with all kinds of vitamins and minerals.

Some vegetables, however, are easier for your blood-sugar mechanisms to deal with than others are. If you had laid off the junk food, chances are you could eat all the vegetables all your days. But you have not. Most of you who are reading this book have done some fairly major damage to your metabolic system already, and need to be careful to choose those vegetables which will tax your body the least. You can eat cucumbers, broccoli, cauliflower, and green beans all day long. You will get sick of them before their few carbs can raise your blood sugar to any great degree.

Potatoes and corn are a different story. Although relatively nutritious, they are best avoided or at the very least indulged in small quantities only occasionally.

The good news is that not only is this diet beneficial to you in respect to blood sugar; it is in fact the healthiest and most natural diet you can eat. Make sure to eat lots of salads and low-carb vegetables, take vitamin supplements, and rejoice in the knowledge that you are doing your body good!

2. How can I live without potatoes? They are such a part of nearly every meal!

There is no getting around it. Giving up potatoes is a major sacrifice. It is particularly difficult to explain when you are at someone's house and pass up the baked potatoes they have prepared, or the scalloped potatoes. In truth there are plenty of other foods that can take the place of potatoes. Americans make potatoes a side dish at almost every meal simply because their parents did before them, and their parents before them. It is not a law of nature or of God. It is a custom.

Experiment. Try things. A large salad will fill you up as easily as a baked potato once did and will provide more vitamins and almost no blood-sugar rise. A dish of cooked cauliflower, a bowl of nuts, or sliced cucumbers will serve. It comes down to this: If you are really serious about living healthy, and avoiding full-blown diabetes and its terrible manifestations, you will consider the potato a small price to pay. No potato is worth your health.

3. What about eating out? How can I stay low-carb in restaurants that feature so many rice, pasta, and potato dishes?

While there are many restaurants that do lean heavily toward pasta and rice dishes, there are almost no restaurants that serve only those kinds of foods. One favorite of mine: At many fancy restaurants they offer a deluxe hamburger with melted cheese that is enormous. I order the hamburger, remove the buns, and eat it as a steak.

It tastes great, costs a lot less than a rib eye, and is quite filling. Add a salad and you have yourself a meal.

At Mexican restaurants, I often order fajitas. I may indulge myself with one fajita wrapped in a tortilla shell (usually these are fairly thin, and one shell is not going to be too many carbs). The rest of the meat I will eat by itself.

Fast-food restaurants are pretty easy to deal with. If it is a hamburger joint, order a hamburger and a salad and remove at least the top bun. Voilà! A low-carb meal. Pizza places are best to avoid. The salad is about the only thing fit to eat. Normal fare at the Subway chain shops is not desirable. Those huge buns are loaded with carbs. If you must eat one of their sandwiches, make sure to remove the top bun. The chips that are always pushed on you are out. Get yourself some peanuts somewhere if you need something more. The good news is that Subway has begun to offer low-carb wraps, which are a vast improvement on their doughy sandwiches. They are truly low in carbs and taste great. They are a little pricey, but hopefully that will change as competition drives prices down.

4. How often should I check my blood-sugar levels?

This depends upon the severity of your condition. If you are a full-fledged diabetic, you should be under a doctor's care, and he or she will tell you how often to check it. If you are experiencing blood-sugar fluctuations, but your doctor has told you that your blood-sugar levels are not at a diabetic level, you have a little more freedom.

It is important that you find out where you are, in

terms of blood-sugar levels. I would advise you to check your blood sugar one to one and a half hours after you finish eating every major meal for about a month, until the picture becomes clear. As you change your diet and begin to exercise, you will almost certainly find your blood-sugar levels returning to a normal, healthy state. If your levels reach 145 or over, you need to rethink the particular meal that led to that. If your fasting blood-sugar levels are over 115 you should see a doctor.

If, by diet, exercise, and weight control, you find that your blood sugar never goes over 135 or 140, and you have lost the jittery hypoglycemic episodes, you should be able to cut down on your blood-sugar testing. When I eat a meal that contains very few carbs there is no reason for me to check my blood sugar. I know it is going to be fine. If I get a little daring, I will want to check it and find out how my body responded. If the reading is too high, I know not to repeat that daring meal again.

One of the best report cards on how you are doing is the fasting blood-sugar level—the reading that you get when you wake up in the morning. If this is under 100 you get an A. If it is a little over, you'd better be a little more strict in your diet. If it is over 120, it is definitely time to see a doctor.

The type 1 diabetic is in a totally different category here. This person must check their blood sugar several times a day. Because they are producing no insulin at all, even a "low-carb" meal can send their blood sugar far too high. They will need to work closely with a doctor all their life and to check their blood sugar constantly. This is not to say that a low-carb diet will do them no good, however. Some are tempted to think, *I have to take insulin anyway—I might as well eat what I like and take a little more insulin to make up for it.* This is a very foolish idea. Though insulin will always be required, there is absolutely no reason to eat loads of carbs and then take huge doses of insulin to make up for it. Insulin is a very needed and useful hormone, but as we've seen, when we flood our bodies with it (either naturally or through shots) as a result of high-carb eating, we do severe damage to our entire physical structure.

5. What about those times when I am at someone's house and simply can't get out of eating foods I know are not good for me?

First of all, this should be an extremely rare occurrence. If you are eating with people that care about you (and who would want to eat with people that don't?) they will understand that you will be eating a little differently than they. However, I will grant that there are occasional times when you find yourself in a situation where you feel you have to eat something that would normally be off your list. In these cases, the rule is this: Take small portions. A tiny piece of strawberry cheesecake is a lot less damaging than a large piece. Don't make the mistake of saying, "I have to eat this; I might as well really have a huge portion and enjoy myself."

I was at a dinner after church one time where they served a very simple meal: spaghetti and salad. I could have simply eaten the salad, but in this case, I decided to have the spaghetti. I simply had a small helping of spaghetti and a large portion of salad.

6. What about occasional cheating?

If you are asking, "Can I?" I can only reply that it's your life and your health. I have to say that I don't cheat much at all. Some people remark about how disciplined I am, but there is something else at work here. I absolutely hate seeing my blood-sugar levels above where they are supposed to be.

Jack Nicklaus once said that he practiced golf shots over and over again until his hands became sore and bloody because he hated the feeling he got from a bad shot. I guess I can kind of identify. Once I learned what kind of foods it took to keep everything on an even keel, I quickly changed my diet to line up with the desired results. It didn't hurt that, as I've mentioned, my mother was a diabetic and had both her legs amputated in the last ten years of her life. In her last few years she wheeled around her house in her wheelchair, but most of her time was spent in her bedroom. It was a lonely, depressing existence, yet to her credit, after an initial period of tears and depression, she found the grace of God sufficient and adjusted to her extremely limited situation. While I admire her spirit, that is one challenge I have no desire to experience. Ordering the salad and passing up the fries is no big deal for me in light of what could easily lie before me.

If you must cheat, the best kind of cheating is planned cheating; the worst is impulse cheating: *That huge slice of pizza looks so good, I just have to indulge!* If you are going to indulge in a high-carb food, plan it well. Make it your plan to have a fairly small portion, and make sure that the rest of the foods you eat at that meal are very low in carbs.

7. What about the rest of my family?

This is an important issue, and one that requires the wisdom of Solomon. If it were just the fact that you require a specialized diet that is totally useless for anyone who doesn't have blood-sugar problems, it would be simple. You could eat your meals and they could have theirs. However, the more you study the benefits of the low-carb diet, the more you will desire to help your loved ones to move toward low-carb eating as well.

There is no one so zealous and so potentially damaging as a new convert. With all your zeal and your desire for your family to be healthy, you cannot go into your kitchen "Carrie Nation"–style with a baseball bat and smash their doughnuts and frozen pizzas. By the time you get to the place where you are solidly in the low-carb camp, you probably will have spent a lot of time and thought on these things. To expect your spouse or your children, who probably do not have blood-sugar problems, and who have not spent any time at all in studying these things (other than listening to you nag them) to immediately change their eating habits is unrealistic and foolish.

First of all, you will need to find a way to make your new lifestyle as gentle on your family as possible. If this means picking up a quarter pounder from McDonald's on nights you know they are having spaghetti, then by all means do it. (Lose the top bun, of course!) Find ways for your loved ones to be supportive of you and not resentful.

If you are blessed with loving and supportive family members, it will make things a whole lot easier. For example, when you have a dish with noodles in it, your spouse can make an extra pot of low-carb noodles. Another idea is to make a meat loaf a little larger than necessary so you can have a couple of lunches out of it afterwards. And it's especially helpful when family members don't gripe about the extra amount of money you sometimes have to spend on low-carb snacks and foods.

Of course you will hopefully not only want your spouse or children to tolerate your diet; you will want to see them embrace healthy patterns of eating as well. Two words of advice: Be gentle and go slow. Don't expect them to change overnight. If they haven't faced the ugly specter of diabetes, they are not likely to have your motivation. If you can steer them away from most sugars and white breads, you are doing well. Remember that grace motivates from the inside. Encourage, inform, and guide, but do not force or expect too much too soon. Look how long it took you to wise up!

8. How about traveling?

Since I travel a lot, this is a question that is near and dear to my heart. Traveling presents hardly any problems at all if 1) you are going to be eating out at restaurants all the time, and 2) you have a definite say in what restaurants you choose. If you are going to be staying with others, you will want to make a few necessary preparations.

First, let the people you will be staying with know about

your diet in advance. I always make sure to tell them that it is for health reasons and share with them how I have suffered from blood-sugar fluctuations in the past. If they merely think that a slim guy like me is trying to stay slim, they are not going to be nearly as tolerant as they will be if they understand I am doing this to keep diabetes at bay.

Second, make sure to bring some low-carb snacks and foods with you. I never go anywhere without a jar of peanut butter and a jar of unsalted peanuts. A bag of low-carb muffins is a great emergency ration. I bought a Tupperware container to carry about a third of a loaf of low-carb bread. It takes a little extra space, but it is well worth it. You may feel foolish bringing your own foods with you, but drop your pride and do it! After you give a short explanation about blood sugar and carbs, they will get over their astonishment and life will go on. If they are having blood-sugar problems of their own, you may do them a world of good.

One great filler snack that I often have is the Wasa cracker with thin sliced chicken and cheese. I bought a miniature cooler, and I use it to keep the chicken and cheese cool on the road. This is a great snack for taking the edge off your hunger and tiding you over until the next meal.

9. What if I am eating a low-carb diet and my blood-sugar levels are still too high?

First, make sure that your meals are truly low-carb. Sometimes one offending food may make an otherwise healthy meal a problem for us.

If you are sure that you are truly eating low-carb and

your blood-sugar levels are high, it is time for you to see your doctor. Your pancreas may be playing out, and producing too little insulin to keep up with even a minimum level of carbs. If so, you may need to take medication or give yourself insulin shots. Even so you will take lower dosages by eating low-carb than you would otherwise, so don't give up on the low-carb diet.

10. What causes the shaky, nervous feeling I get when I eat a meal high in carbs and then go a while without eating?

The odd thing is, when you are feeling those shaky feelings your blood sugar is actually too low—as a result of your blood sugar being too high about an hour or two ago! The high-carb meal was more than your body could easily handle. In your younger days, your more efficient metabolism could have dealt with these carbs quickly. Your pancreas would have released a small amount of insulin, your receptor cells would have made use of that insulin and rapidly dispatched the carbs and brought the blood-sugar levels to normal.

Today your pancreas is still producing the insulin, but your metabolism just isn't what it used to be. To make up for this, your pancreas gamely produces prodigious amounts of insulin, which helps, but it takes time for the receptor cells to use the insulin and lower the blood sugar. Finally the blood sugar comes down, but there is a large amount of "leftover insulin" hanging around your bloodstream with nothing to do. The excess insulin now begins to drive your blood-sugar down lower and lower, but there are no carbs left for it to deal with. As a result, your blood sugar goes far too low. As it drops you begin to feel strange. Your body is telling you that things are not right. Shakiness and nervousness are often experienced. If your blood sugar gets too low, you could pass out or even die.

Few people get to this level, but it can happen. For most, the shakiness and nervousness are all they will experience for a period of time, until their pancreas finally begins to give out. As that happens the insulin level decreases, and the blood-sugar levels increase. Often high blood sugar will not give as clear a signal to your body as low blood sugar, and so you may feel that things have straightened out and all is well. In truth you are entering the world of full-blown diabetes. While you are having those shaky feelings, now is the time to do something about your diet and your lifestyle. There is still hope for you. Your pancreas is working fine, but your metabolism is falling behind. Be kind to your overworked pancreas and make those dietary and lifestyle changes now!

11. Isn't it possible to have hypoglycemia for several decades and never develop diabetes?

It is indeed possible. An older woman I know well has struggled with hypoglycemia for the last 20 years (she's 80 at the time of writing) and it has never developed into diabetes. This is one of those mysteries that has its answer in genetics. Along the same lines there are people who are overweight, are couch potatoes, eat sweets like crazy all their lives, and never develop diabetes. There are people in certain ethnic groups, such as American Indians and Hispanics, that develop diabetes at far greater rates than those of Northern European heritage. We don't know all the reasons for this. All I can say is that if you have hypoglycemic symptoms you are at a much greater risk for diabetes than if you do not. You might be able to get through life and never develop diabetes, but there is a pretty fair chance that you won't. Why take a chance? Also, that high-carb, low-exercise way of life might well kill you prematurely through a heart attack or stroke. What is the advantage of dying at 50 of a heart attack even though you may have somehow avoided diabetes?

12. Why shouldn't I just trust God to heal me and forget the exercise and diet?

This is a question that not many would ask, and so if this has been on your mind I commend you for considering the possibility of divine healing. I would agree that God can and does heal in spectacular ways, without any medical means whatsoever. If you want to believe God for such a healing, far be it from me to discourage you.

Having said that, let me also make this point. Whether God heals you this way or not, the truth is that a high-carb, high-sugar diet is a form of self-abuse. And when you live a physically inactive life you are making poor use of one of God's special gifts: your body. (It may be hard for you to think of your body as a gift, but believe me, it is. What would you do without it?) Therefore, having gained the knowledge you now have, you will need to make some changes in your lifestyle, divine healing or not. And who is to say that God isn't answering your prayer for divine healing by showing you the principles of low-carb eating, exercise, and weight control?

13. *Are my kids at any risk of blood-sugar problems now, or will they need to reach middle age before they face these things?*

Sad to say, children are being ravaged by diabetes today in America at rates never seen before. This is, no doubt, due to the unprecedented levels of obesity among children, physical inactivity as a result of TV, computers, and video games, and a high-carb onslaught that has actually been endorsed by many medical professionals. The older term for type 2 diabetes, "adult onset diabetes," is becoming a misnomer because of so many children coming down with this terrible affliction.

Every responsible parent needs to take steps to protect their children. While you don't necessarily have to take away all sweets, at least make candy and sodas a treat rather than a given at every meal and every day. Serve so many salads to your kids that they will begin to like them out of self-defense if nothing else. Cut back considerably on white bread products. Talk to them about what carbs can do to their bloodstream. Plan tasty low-carb meals frequently. Make rolls and biscuits the exception rather than the rule. Establish them in positive eating habits while they are young—and when they get old, hopefully they will not depart from them.

14. *Can diabetes be reversed?*

Apart from miraculous healing, there is still great hope for those who suffer from diabetes. One group did a study of 14 Australian aborigines who had moved to the United States and developed diabetes over time.[8] The researchers paid the way for these men to go back to Australia and live as they had formerly lived before coming to America. This involved a radical change in diet, with almost all sweets and white breads being eliminated. Within a few weeks these men, whose blood-sugar levels had registered clearly in the diabetic range, were now showing normal blood sugar. Interestingly, the dietary change was their only change. They were not getting all that much more exercise than in America. So were these men diabetics or not? It would appear that the answer to that question lay in where they were and what they ate. You might sum up their situation by saying that they had the potential for diabetes, had the predisposition for diabetes, but didn't have to have diabetes or its symptoms as long as they watched what they ate.

So it is with most type 2 diabetics, as well as those who are in the hypoglycemic pre-diabetic stage. Break enough of your Creator's laws and you will sure enough become diabetic. Walk in wisdom and you can avoid diabetes for 10 years, 20 years, and in many cases the rest of your life.

By eating a low-carb diet, maintaining a proper weight, and exercising 40 minutes five to six days a week, most people who have had blood sugar problems, including those whose levels have reached the diabetes classification, can keep their blood sugar under control. I am one of those. I do not consider myself to be a diabetic. I do realize that I have passed up a marvelous chance to become diabetic!

15. *Should I try to avoid red meat as much as possible?*

The research that has been done on the Atkins diet

indicates that red meat, eaten in the context of a low-carb diet, is not the problem that the low-fat, high-carb gurus have made it out to be. As long as you keep your carbs low, you can enjoy hamburger meat, steaks, and meat loaf without guilt. That having been said, the principle of moderation should always be a part of your life. Don't just eat red meat alone; eat fish, chicken, and turkey as well. The sensible approach here is don't be afraid of red meat, but don't just load up on it either. The real danger is for the person who eats lots of red meat and lots of high-carb foods. They are asking for trouble—and chances are they will get it.

16. How can I get low-carb products?

At present most low-carb products can be purchased either in health-food stores or on the Internet. Atkins.com is a great source for almost everything, although they charge a standard $7.50 fee for any order, whether a $5 muffin mix or a $200 combined order. Go to a search engine and type in "low-carb products," and you should have no trouble finding several choices.

Health-food stores are beginning to carry a few low-carb products, but the selection is often limited. Usually they specialize in shakes, low-carb bars, and muffin mixes. As the low-carb diet becomes more and more popular look for this to change. You can find a surprising number of low-carb items at the larger grocery stores. Low-carb bread can often be found among the other breads. Go to the specialty food sections, and you can often find low-carb jellies and ketchup, Splenda, and quite a number of other items.

I would start by ordering a catalog from several of the larger low-carb companies. This will give you a good idea of what is out there, and then you can check other sources for similar products. Keep in mind that there are loads of low-carb recipes to be found on the Internet, made with "regular" foods. Do some research and experimenting, and you can add to your low-carb repertoire. The key thing is to realize that the foods you need are out there. It may take a little work to find them and a little extra money to add them to your shopping list, but they are one of the best investments in your health you can make.

More and more low-carb products are becoming available. The choices and options are greater now than they have ever been. We are blessed!

17. Do I really have to give up all fruits?

No, you do not have to give up on fruit. But you will need to be careful and wise in your eating of fruit. The lower-carb fruits are the ones you should emphasize in your diet—melons and berries being the best. Small tangerines are an excellent source of vitamin C that are actually lower in carbs than most. The worst way to take fruit is through fruit juice. Here you are getting a high concentration of sugar that has been released from its house of fiber. Thus the sugar hits your bloodstream hard and fast—as your glucomoter will faithfully testify. The higher-carb fruits (bananas, apples, and large oranges being examples) should be taken sparingly and in half portions divided over two meals, rather than all at once.

18. I have started on the low-carb diet, and I feel as though I have less energy than before. Is it really good for me to do without carbs and the energy they provide?

First of all, you are not supposed to "do without carbs." I cannot emphasize this enough: What you need is a low-carb diet, not a no-carb diet. It is true that carbs can provide energy, but the energy they provide is deceptive. They give you an immediate boost as your blood-sugar levels ratchet up, but this will soon lead to a precipitous drop in blood sugar and the consequent feelings of weakness and hunger. It is truly a vicious cycle. I personally have never felt a loss of energy from my low-carb lifestyle, although I have heard of some that have. This is probably because my diet changed gradually. As I learned more and more about what foods my body could tolerate, I adjusted my diet accordingly and never experienced some of the physical trauma that occurs when you go from one diet to another "cold turkey."

I am convinced that much of the "weakness" reported by new low-carbers is nothing more than the body responding to a different dietary regime. Give yourself time and it will probably pass. I can eat a low-carb breakfast of eggs, bacon, and a low-carb muffin, and then spend a vigorous 40 minutes huffing, puffing, and sweating on the treadmill, and feel absolutely euphoric afterwards. I'm not saying I don't feel some tiredness (a brisk three-mile walk has a way of doing that!), but it feels so great to know I have done my body a world of good. I travel, preach, teach, write, tape television programs, and fulfill all the responsibilities of my ministry without any feelings of weakness. So it is hard for me to give too much credence to the idea that the only way you can engage in vigorous physical activity is to "load up on the carbs."

19. How can I convince my family and friends I'm not a fanatic?

The main thing here is to talk frankly about your blood-sugar problems and what you have discovered. As long as your friends realize that you are eating differently due to health difficulties, they will be understanding. If you give them the impression that you are just doing this to be fashionably slim or are on the verge of becoming anorexic, they will be concerned or put off. Use the "D" word (diabetes) and let them know that you are determined by God's grace not to be a victim of this terrible plague. One of the blessings you will receive from being frank is that almost for sure you will run across others that are also struggling with runaway blood sugar, and may be God's means for their healing. Lend or give them this book. It just might change their life and their future!

CHAPTER 12

Going the Distance

You have done it! You have made major changes in your diet, reducing your carbohydrate intake significantly, you have established a solid exercise program, and your blood-sugar levels have stabilized. The ugly specter of diabetes is retreating fast, and you couldn't be happier!

Now, what about the next 30-plus years? As with diet and nearly everything else, it is easier to achieve a goal than it is to maintain it. And maintain it you must. Day by day, month by month, and year by year you are going to need to practice what you have learned for decades, if God grants—and assuming you aren't 90 already!

I have said it before, but I cannot say it enough: lifestyle, lifestyle, lifestyle. You have not gone on a temporary diet to "fix" something. You have not begun a little exercise program just to get you over the hump, then to go back to your old ways. The old has died, the new has come! Any changes you cannot make for a lifetime are not worth making at all. In fact they will cause you more harm than good, in that your repeated failures will cement your inertia and leave you helpless and hopeless.

In order to facilitate a lifetime of good metabolic behavior, there are a few keys that I want to share with you.

Enjoyment Is Crucial

First, be creative with your meals. Search the Internet and various low-carb books for recipes that suit you. Try out anything that sounds good until you find a diet varied enough and tasty enough that you can say, "This, I can live with for a lifetime." Of course all meats are "fair game" (pun intended) and that helps a lot! Rib eyes, T-bones, sirloins, chicken in all kinds of ways, fish galore (without the breading), veal, and so forth can make for the foundation of a great meal. There are infinite varieties in fixing these meats, so plunge in and enjoy.

Enjoy sweets now and then. I still haven't lost my sweet tooth, and I am thrilled that there are so many different ways I can satisfy that tooth and still keep to my low-carb regimen. I have even found ice-cream bars sweetened with Splenda that have only six net carbs each. I have one of these bars with my coffee at night, toss in a few peanuts, and I'm a happy guy. One of my absolute favorites is a cheesecake with low-carb chocolate drizzled over the top and an almond crust on the bottom. It is awesome!* (Remember, this can't be an ordinary cheese-cake. Make sure it is from a low-carb recipe.)

What I'm saying here is that all the joy and the pleasure of eating does not get up and leave when you alter your diet and reduce your carbohydrates. There are still wonderful foods to be eaten, great desserts to enjoy, and many culinary pleasures that await you. This is vitally important to realize and take advantage of, because if you limit yourself to a few dull items, day after day, you will never make it. Sooner or later your taste buds will rebel and you'll end up going down to the local Dairy Queen for a hot-fudge sundae or a Blizzard. So don't deprive yourself unnecessarily. Do your homework, find meals and desserts that please you, and create for yourself a lifestyle that you can live with for the next 30 or 40 years.

Sacrifices and Substitutes

You will, of course, be making some sacrifices. When you go out to eat with someone who orders a baked potato drenched in butter, sour cream, and bacon bits you may find yourself asking, "What have I gotten myself into?" (The answer, of course, is health!) One of the things that will help you make the necessary sacrifices is to see your lifestyle as a prescription written for you from your Creator. God in His great love for you has shown you what you need to do to be healthy. Whatever your friends may eat, whatever indulgences they may allow themselves, you are under "doctor's orders."

Be sure to take advantage of the many substitutes that are available. You may have to make sacrifices, but there

---

* See appendix C for this recipe and others.

is no need to make any more sacrifices than necessary. When my family has tacos, I have a taco as well. I just use a low-carb shell and eat without guilt or runaway blood sugar. On those days when I allow myself rice, I always have brown rice rather than white, and take a somewhat smaller helping than I would have in the old days. If we are having a meal where bread seems the natural side dish, I don't do without. I have a tasty low-carb muffin. There is low-carb ketchup for my meat loaf, low-carb barbecue sauce when I barbecue pork steaks, and even low-carb pancake syrup on my low-carb pancakes. I may not eat as wide a diet as I did before my blood-sugar problems, but I eat a whole lot more varied menu than when I first began to cut carbs and didn't know about these things.

Stay current on low-carb news, research, and books. The more you understand the principles of nutrition, the more motivated you will be to stay true to your diet. Read Dr. Atkins' books and other solid books on the power of low-carb eating. The Bible says that, in the way a person "thinks in his heart, so he is" (Proverbs 23:7). What you think on will determine what you do and what you become. And for those who need some help in the area of blood sugar, read books like *Protein Power* by Michael Eades, *Dr. Atkins' New Diet Revolution* by Robert Atkins, *Beat Diabetes* by Margaret Blackstone, and *Diabetes Solution* by Richard Bernstein (especially helpful for type 1 diabetics). Don't just read these all at once and then forget it. Read them periodically, and find other books that promote low-carb living. Check out low-carb web-sites and subscribe to low-carb e-mail newsletters. Keep in touch with this area of knowledge and you'll not lag in motivation!

Another means of staying true to your new lifestyle is to share with others the deliverance you have found. You don't realize it, but there are people all through your world who are having serious blood-sugar problems—diabetics and borderline diabetics who don't have a clue as to what they can do to find a remedy. Many people are so afraid of even the word *diabetes* that they will put off having themselves checked by a doctor for fear of what they might find. Ignorance and fear are best friends. Where you find one you will almost always find the other.

Finally, you will find that the sacrifices you make will be a lot easier when you take the time to count your blessings. The fact that you are "not like other people" can be depressing, especially when you see them eating french-silk pie and you say, "No, thank you—I don't eat sugar," for the umpteenth time. When that happens, remind yourself that you really are blessed. When you consider the blessings of family and friends, of church and healthy activities, of so many of the simple pleasures of life, doing without sugar, pasta, bread, and potatoes is a very tiny thing. So what if you have to make a few sacrifices for two or three decades? In comparison to all that your Creator has provided, you have nothing to complain about.

As You Grow Older

Regardless of your age, the fact is that you will never be younger than you are at this present moment. And with aging come some not-so-pleasant realities.

Because diabetes and blood-sugar troubles are so entwined with our metabolism, aging is not the friend of the diabetic or the pre-diabetic. Your body is not as fast as it was, your reflexes aren't as quick, but more to the point, your metabolism isn't as efficient.

A poorly functioning metabolism is the foundation for blood-sugar problems. The type 1 diabetic's problems stem from a malfunctioning pancreas, but for the type 2, the pancreas may work just great until it finally gives out from overwork because of a body that can't process sugar anymore.

To use a metaphor, diabetes is a vicious enemy that lurks outside your campfire waiting for the fires of your metabolism to burn low. When the fires burn too low your enemy will strike hard and fast, and you will hardly know what hit you. Your task, then, is to keep the fires burning as bright as possible as long as possible. Our goal is to keep diabetes at bay for as long as we can. Every year without diabetes is a blessing, a decade without it is a wonder, and to spend your remaining years without it and die of old age (if God grants) is the best of all!

If you fail to attain the full goal but do, in fact, push diabetes 10 to 15 years away, you have achieved a great thing. What price can you put on 15 years of good health? I personally believe that for most potential type 2 diabetics (like me), it should be possible to live our entire lives with normal blood-sugar levels—and without pills or shots. Of course, be checked by a doctor and keep close tabs on your fasting blood-sugar level. But be encouraged that living without diabetes is not only possible but likely if you will follow the Creator's design.

And even if you fail to prevent diabetes altogether, by following the dietary, exercise, and weight control guidelines, the diabetic symptoms will be far less severe than they otherwise would be, and your ability to control your blood-sugar levels will be greatly enhanced. In short, you really cannot afford not to do everything you can to minimize the effect of this diabolical enemy upon your life.

As you age, your body's ability to handle sugar will deteriorate. This happens with nearly everyone but is far more pronounced with those who have diabetic tendencies. The response you make to your body's weakening ability to process sugar will make a big difference in which of these categories you find yourself in. Here are some of the changes you can make as you move from middle age to your later years.

Weight

Because weight (and fat) makes such a big difference in how efficiently you can handle carbohydrates and glucose, it makes sense that you want to be on the lean side of things from the moment that you first notice diabetic symptoms. As you age, and your metabolism slows down, and your body loses its youthful efficiency, you will do yourself a favor by becoming leaner still. Obviously you don't want to become a walking skeleton; that would definitely not be helpful. But you do want to give yourself a fighting chance by staying slim.

It may be necessary to drop five or ten pounds more than you were able to successfully carry in younger years. At this point you definitely do not want to be one pound over the recommended weight for your height and bone structure. Consider shedding a few more pounds and keeping them off as an antidote to your body's aging process. You especially do not want to have any kind of "paunch" around your middle at this stage. That is deadly for people with diabetic tendencies at any age, and all the more so as you move into your latter years.

Exercise

As you age your exercise needs and abilities are going to change, and you will need to adjust accordingly. If you have been jogging, there will likely come a time when jogging is no longer appropriate for you, as your knees begin to wear, and soreness becomes more than an occasional visitor. You will probably need to make your exercise sessions less intense but longer. By your 60s most people will probably come to a point where a good, brisk walk (or a swim when possible) is better than the more intense activities like jogging, tennis, basketball, and so forth.

Make sure your walks don't become too leisurely, however. Walk fast enough to get your heart pumping a little faster than normal, and your blood circulating freely. Also, since you are now exercising less strenuously, you will need to exercise for a slightly longer period of time. This usually works out fine, as by this time you are either retired or getting closer to retirement. An hour of brisk walking is about right. As I mentioned previously, the morning is by far the better time to exercise. You will not only get your metabolism cranked up after your body has been on pause all night long, but you will ensure that no amount of busyness later on in the day prevents you from your exercise time.

Regardless of your age you will need to exercise. This

is better than any medicine on the market for bringing blood-sugar levels in line, and is just too valuable to ignore. Change your schedule if you need to, alter your particular exercises, but don't give up! You need to work your body, and this will never change!

Diet

As with exercise, diet may need to be altered in your golden years. Be sure and keep a sharp eye on your blood-sugar levels. If you find your fasting blood-sugar level rising in spite of regular exercise and staying on the slim side, you will probably need to be a little more strict in your intake of carbohydrates. Cut back a little more on the fruits, the brown rice, and other larger sources of carbs until you see those levels where they need to be.

At no time will you ever want to do away with carbohydrates altogether! All through this book I have preached the low-carb lifestyle to you, but I would never tell you to try to do without any carbs. That would be most foolish and could cause more problems than it helps. Occasional whole-wheat crackers, brown rice, and other foods a little on the high-carb side are needed by your body for energy and other vital functions.

Watch your carbs, watch your blood-sugar, and cut back a little more in your older years if necessary. Be sure and continue to take vitamin supplements as part of your daily regimen. These will help you to have a potent immune system and make you far less liable to other sicknesses and diseases.

The Thrill of Winning

I like to win. I always have. When my wife and I were dating, we went to my old elementary school field to throw a football around. We ran across three junior high boys who were also tossing a football. Somehow or other we ended up in a game against each other. With my competitive nature I quickly got into the spirit of the game and started directing my wife-to-be in intricate pass patterns and tricky running plays. After a little while it dawned on her just how much this little game meant to me. She looked at me in surprise and said, "You really want to win, don't you?"

I forget exactly what I said at that point, but if I had been completely honest I would have said something like, "Well, of course I want to win. What's the use of playing if we're not going to play to win?" That has always been my attitude. And while it is possible to push competition beyond the bounds of righteousness, it is generally a pretty good attitude to hold, especially when you are in a fight for your life.

And that is exactly what runaway blood sugar is. The monster of diabetes is lurking nearby. It wants to spoil your most beautiful moments, disrupt the natural process of aging, ruin your golden years, and lop off a decade or more from your allotted time.

Diabetes will not be impressed with gentle, mild efforts. A few token modifications of lifestyle will not be enough. You might as well try putting out a forest fire with a few tablespoons of water. You will only be kidding yourself.

You must have a reason for good health. That sounds silly, I know. After all isn't good health itself reason enough? Sadly the answer is no, it is not. Many people find themselves so miserable in their latter years that they don't care whether they live or die, whether they are sick or well. They are so emotionally unhealthy that physical problems don't seem all that significant.

So walk with God. Take an interest in others. Develop relationships. Volunteer your time for noble causes. Be active in your church. Indulge fully in *life!* As you do, you will have more to live for than merely yourself. There will be people who need you, people who won't do so well if you are sick or dead. Your interest in life will be like medicine in itself. It will give you the motivation to invest time and energy in staying healthy for the glory of God and the good of others.

Embrace this new season of your life. You may not run as fast or hit a golf ball as far, but you can gain wisdom far beyond the years of your youth. So what if you have to think about fish-oil supplements or take readings of your blood-sugar levels to see how you are doing! Big deal!

The Best Source of Motivation

You are not alone. If you are a Christian, God is your Resource. His power, His love—and yes, His knowledge of how our bodies work—are available to those who seek. Health may be elusive and may not be an instant work, but dare to believe that there is a pathway to health for you. You have friends in high places!

You have a loving Father and a caring Savior who are ready to jump into your situation and provide some very tangible help. It may never have occurred to you just how prominent healing is in the Bible. In the Old Testament He declared to Israel, "I am the Lord that healeth thee"

(Exodus 15:26). He gave them dietary and sanitary laws, and promised that if they would keep His commandments, there would be no sickness or even miscarriages among them (Exodus 23:25-26). Clearly God was concerned with the health of His people.

This concern didn't end with the conclusion of the Old Testament. During the days of Jesus, healing was one of the most prominent features of His ministry. He healed people "en masse." He healed constantly. He refused no one who came to Him.

After Jesus' resurrection, His disciples carried on this healing ministry. Peter's shadow brought healing; Paul's handkerchiefs brought healing. James counseled the sick to "call for the elders of the church, and let them pray over him...and the prayer of faith shall save the sick" (James 5:14-15).

With all the abundant scriptural evidence for healing, it shouldn't be too much of a stretch for us to consider that just maybe God doesn't expect us to merely accept sickness as His sovereign will for our lives and refuse to ever pray for health or hope to be healthy!

Then Why Did God Give Me This Problem?

Before we talk more about motivation, let's talk about an issue that troubles some Christians. With healing so prominent in the Bible, they ask, why did God give me this blood-sugar condition in the first place?

I will start by saying that I don't believe God did give you this condition—at least not in the sense that many would mean. I do not believe that God is up in heaven with a diabetes gun zapping people with this terrible affliction for reasons only He knows.

God has created our world with myriads of causes and effects. He does not need to take extraordinary measures to bring about effects from causes. For example, people who constantly force cigarette smoke into their lungs are much more likely to contract lung cancer than those who don't. This doesn't mean God is striking them with cancer; it means they are breaking physical laws and experiencing the consequences of their actions.

So it is with diabetes. There are cultures in the world where diabetes is unknown. Does this mean that God loves those people more than Americans? Of course not. It simply means that with our typical American lifestyle of inactivity, obesity, and stuffing ourselves with tons of white flour and sugar, we have made ourselves susceptible to this terrible condition.

God is for you, though! He wants you well. He sent His Son as a Savior to the world, and as Jesus walked throughout Israel He had the amazing habit of healing all the sick who came to Him. The Bible says of Him,

> God anointed Jesus of Nazareth with the Holy Spirit and power, who went about doing good, healing all who were oppressed by the devil, for God was with Him (Acts 10:38).

Jesus

In all the struggles of life, then, it is vital that we see Jesus is the object of our faith. Every good gift can truly be said to come from God, but He gives those gifts through His Son and calls upon us to focus our faith upon Him. Thus we do not merely declare that we trust God as our Savior; we freely acknowledge that God's Son, Jesus Christ, is a Savior to us. We look to God as our Deliverer, but know that His deliverance comes through Jesus. The person who declares His trust in God but never acknowledges any faith in Jesus has not trusted in God at all. The apostle John writes,

> Whoever denies the Son does not have the
> Father either; he who acknowledges the Son
> has the Father also (1 John 2:23).

We see Jesus exalted in every role that God exercises toward suffering humanity. Jesus is our Redeemer, Savior, Healer, Teacher, Life-Giver, and on and on and on. Those who abide in Jesus and grow in His grace will continually discover new dimensions of their Lord. With each succeeding victory of faith, their confidence in Him will mount higher and higher.

As a Christian, your struggle with blood sugar is more than a matter of carbohydrates, insulin, and insulin-receptor cells. Every physical battle has a spiritual component. Yes, there are physical principles to discover and employ, but there is more, far more. We have a Resource the world knows nothing about. Jesus is mighty to save. Approach the throne of grace with confidence. Obey the physical laws He reveals to you, but look to Him to take you places that diet and exercise alone could never take you. Trust Him for a lifetime of victory over diabetes and blood-sugar woes. Look to Him as the source of your motivation for maintaining a healthy lifestyle for the rest of your days. He is faithful.

The Holy Spirit

Jesus told us that those who would believe on Him for salvation would be given the gift of the Holy Spirit:

> "Whoever believes in me, as the Scripture has said, streams of living water will flow from within him." By this he meant the Spirit (John 7:38-39 NIV).

Christians have a resource that non-Christians do not. The Holy Spirit fulfills many, many roles in the life of the believer. He leads us into all truth, brings to our remembrance the words of Jesus, empowers us to witness, and gives us supernatural gifts to demonstrate the glory of God. One of the major roles He plays has to do with motivation. During the Old Testament era, God told Israel to keep His laws and they would be life to them. Israel had great intentions and often made vows to be God's people, to keep His laws, and to maintain His covenant. But they had no power to keep those good intentions.

I'm going to let you in on a secret. God knew that they would fail all along. He wasn't surprised. He was grieved, but He was not surprised. The human will is a marvelous thing, but it has been spoiled by original sin. As in Paul's classic description in Romans 7, we do those things we hate, and those things we want to do we fail to do. With all the threats of punishment for lawbreakers and promises of reward for obedience, Israel still failed miserably.

God used Israel to show the human race a powerful truth. By the strength of our wills we will always come up short. But God did not leave us to merely contemplate Israel's failure and dwell on our own similar fate. He made some incredible promises to His people, promises that are fulfilled whenever we place our faith unreservedly in His Son, Jesus Christ. Listen to what He declares through Ezekiel:

> I will give them one heart, and I will put a new spirit within them, and take the stony heart out of their flesh, and give them a heart of flesh, that they may walk in My statutes and keep My judgments and do them; and they shall be My people, and I will be their God (Ezekiel 11:19-20).

God is declaring that He will give Israel such a powerful inner motivation that keeping His laws and His commandments will no longer be a problem for them. He will see to it Himself! The way He accomplishes this is through the Holy Spirit. Israel will no longer be motivated by the whip and the carrot; they will be motivated by the indwelling God, constantly pumping new life and righteous desires into them. They *will* walk in His statues and keep His judgments. Then this promise is repeated in Hebrews 10 in reference to Christians, God's New Testament people.

Christ in You

Every genuine Christian has more than enough motivational drive within them to live right, eat right, exercise, and live free from any and every form of addiction. The most motivated individual who ever walked the earth was the Lord Jesus. He was so highly motivated that He never sinned one time. His whole life was consumed with doing the will of God. The Messianic psalm, in describing Jesus' attitude toward morality, declared, "You love righteousness and hate wickedness; therefore God, Your God, has anointed You with the oil of gladness more than Your companions" (Psalm 45:7).

Wouldn't it be wonderful if we could have this kind of motivation in our lives? Here's a secret few Christians seem to realize: We do! When one is born again, he receives the very nature of Christ, in the Person of the Holy Spirit. This is why the Bible talks about "Christ in you." We have His love for righteousness, His hatred of sin, His self-control, His intense desire for the will of God. And yes, we have His ability to eat, drink, and exercise to the glory of God. (You say that you can't imagine our Lord doing push-ups! He probably didn't. But if we walked as many miles as He did, we could skip all other forms of exercise as well.)

Before you ever start this program to conquer blood-sugar problems, commit everything to God in prayer. Let Jesus know that He is your Shepherd and that you trust Him to lead you through every difficulty. Acknowledge your own weakness, but be just as quick to acknowledge His strength. Trust Him to make you to "will and to do for His good pleasure." Don't just do this at the beginning, however. Continue to confess Christ as your Strength, your Healer, and your Deliverer. Expect Him to keep you faithful in spite of your weakness. Don't merely beg Him to do it; trust Him to do it, and don't let a day go by where you don't thank Him for giving you the victory.

Salvation is "by grace through faith." This is not only true for salvation from sin, which gives us eternal life. This is also true for more temporal salvations. Your "salvation" from blood sugar will be by grace through faith. Confess Christ as your Savior from diabetes, just as you do your Savior from sin and hell. He will be to you what you acknowledge Him to be. This is not merely a matter of semantics. This is life or death, victory or defeat. As you look to Jesus, He will not only go to work in changing your body, He will also release a powerful river of motivation that will keep you true to those principles of eating and living that will serve you well all of your days. As you walk in victory, Jesus will receive the glory, and that is exactly as it should be.

God, the Ultimate Behavior-Changer

Behavior change is God's specialty. He loves to provide the spiritual power to radically change people for the better. He has been doing this a long time and He is very, very good at what He does. He is eager to help you get control of your appetites. If you will ask Him, and trust Him, the outcome is absolutely sure.

Romans chapter 6 is the Christian's "emancipation proclamation" from slavery to sin. Take a look at these sample verses:

- Verse 6: "Our old man was crucified with Him, that the body of sin might be done away with, that we should no longer be slaves of sin."

- Verse 11: "Reckon yourselves to be dead indeed to sin, but alive to God in Christ Jesus our Lord."

- Verse 14: "Sin shall not have dominion over you, for you are not under law but under grace."

- Verse 18: "Having been set free from sin, you became slaves of righteousness."

Be sure and read and meditate on your emancipation frequently. Thank God again and again that you are dead to sin and alive to Him. You can be sure you're on solid ground in saying this, for that is exactly what the Word of God tells us!

As you do this you will be changing inwardly. You will experience an ever-increasing release of the Spirit's power in this area of your life. Jesus was your Deliverer all along. When you confess Him you do not make Him so. Yet as you confess and acknowledge Him thus, you will begin to live in the benefits of that deliverance. Yes, there will be things for you to do, and yes, there will be sacrifices to be made, but the victory will ultimately be won through faith in our mighty Savior. Never forget that!

Final Thoughts

As you share the story of how God provided you deliverance, and the joy of seeing the Goliath of diabetes slain at your feet, you will be encouraging others to investigate and find deliverance for themselves. As people ask you why you eat the way you do (and they will surely ask you), it is a perfect opportunity to share your "testimony." And it really is a testimony. You were in desperate straits, and God heard your prayer and delivered you. Deliverance is God's business—and it is a blessing for people to hear about it.

Trust God to give you all it takes to preserve your whole spirit, soul, and body blameless until the coming of Christ. Let your prayers reflect your faith and nourish your faith. Start your mornings by thanking Jesus for being your Shepherd to lead you through the day. Thank Him for keeping you from indulging in foods that you know you must not eat. If you will trust Him, He will surely do His part.

The same grace that led you to Christ in the first place is leading you to victory over excess blood sugar. That grace that began your spiritual life will be with you all through your years. Jesus, your Good Shepherd, will lead you through your 40s, 50s, 60s, 70s…He will lead you on this earth as long as He deems fit for you to serve Him here.

'Tis grace that brought me safe thus far,
and grace will lead me home.

Sample Meals

There are lots of low-carb recipes and meal plans available—and I am no chef, so I'm not going to give you an extensive list of recipes and fancy meals for you to try. I am a pretty basic guy, so I don't venture nearly as far as others, who are constantly on a quest for new and exciting low-carb sensations. But I will give you a week's worth of low-carb meals made up of simple things that nearly every American will be familiar with, just to give you an idea of how to get started. For you with a more exotic palate, buy some books and do some research on the Internet. The sky's the limit!

Sunday

Breakfast:

Low-carb cereal with a low-carb milk substitute

Wasa cracker with two slices of sliced chicken breast and slice of cheese

Lunch:

McDonald's double cheeseburger minus the top bun

Side salad with ranch dressing

Handful of peanuts

Supper:

Peanut-butter-and-jelly sandwich using low-carb bread and low-carb jelly

Bowl of cottage cheese

Piece of beef jerky or other meat I can find in the refrigerator

Monday

Breakfast:

Two fried eggs

Bacon or sausage

Slice of low-carb bread, toasted and with low-carb jelly on it

Lunch:

Two Wasa crackers with Swanson Chicken breast in water (comes in a can like tuna) made into a "tuna salad sandwich"–like spread

Low-carb yogurt (you can buy this or make your own using plain yogurt and adding berries)

Supper:

One or two fajitas served on (in) low-carb tortilla shells

Salad with any dressing of choice, except sugary ones like french or thousand island

Bowl of broccoli with melted cheese on top

Tuesday

Breakfast:

Wasa cracker with two slices of chicken breast (or turkey) and one slice of cheese of choice

Two slices of cantaloupe

Lunch:

Chef salad with lettuce, chicken strips, cheese, broccoli, cauliflower, and green peppers

Supper:

Meat loaf

Bowl of cauliflower with melted cheese on top

Green beans

Low-carb muffin

Wednesday

Breakfast:

Egg omelet, with ham, cheese, onions, and green peppers

Low-carb bagel with melted cheese on top and low-carb jelly if desired

Lunch:

Meat loaf (left over from last night)

Celery stalk with peanut butter

Small tangerine (surprisingly, only about eight grams of carbs)

Supper:

Fish fillet (frozen type baked in oven, not breaded)

Salad

Smaller portion of brown rice

Green beans

Thursday

Breakfast:

Low-carb hot cereal

Piece of cheese

Lunch:

Taco on low-carb tortilla

Cottage cheese and peaches (peach slices come from half of a "real" peach, not the syrupy peach slices from a can!)

Low-carb muffin

Supper:

Salmon patty

Salad

Celery with cream cheese

Tomato slices

Friday

Breakfast:

Scrambled eggs

Ham

Tomato slices (left over from last night)

Lunch:

Salmon patty (left over from last night)

Medium portion of barbecued beans (not the sweetened kind)

Wasa cracker with cream cheese

Supper:

Barbecued chicken using low-carb barbecue sauce

Salad

Low-carb muffin

Bowl of strawberries (eight to ten medium-sized)

Saturday

Breakfast:

Low-carb pancakes (three to four) with low-carb syrup

Two sausages

Lunch:

Lunch-meat sandwich (on low-carb bread) with tomato slice and cheese

Bowl of cottage cheese and raspberries

Nuts of your choosing

Supper:

   Roast beef

   Salad

   Dill pickle (cucumbers and pickles have almost no carbs;
      eat as many as you want)

   Wasa cracker with cream cheese

I know this diet is pretty basic, and there are certainly a lot of other options for creative minds to explore. This is just to get you started with one week of simple low-carb eating. If you have been checking your blood-sugar levels and are making the change from the standard American diet to this one, you should see a dramatic drop in your blood-sugar readings. If you are on medication, keep close watch on your blood sugar. Chances are you won't need as much medication as before.

It won't be difficult to modify this plan to suit your personal preferences. Almost any meat can be substituted for any other. Meat has so few carbs in it that it is hardly worth noticing. Yes, you can eat too much meat—but on the other hand, you shouldn't be afraid of it either. (Be careful, however, of meats that are coated with bread coatings such as fish or chicken. These coatings can radically jack up the number of carbs and turn meat into a major source of carbs. Many of the frozen fish portions you find in the stores have heavy bread coatings and are not at all good for people with blood-sugar problems.)

The Really Good Stuff

As I have searched for great recipes and low-carb products, I have run across a few real gems that make my life much more pleasant. These foods are so great-tasting that I just had to share them in a special section with you. Enjoy!

Low-Carb Pancakes

Being a rigid traditionalist, I have been eating a Saturday-morning breakfast of pancakes and sausage nearly all of my life. When I realized that those doughy, white-flour pancakes, drenched in sugary syrup, were wreaking havoc with my blood sugar, I knew they would

207

have to go. I soon discovered low-carb pancake mixes that were available in health-food stores and through the Internet. But the taste! It was enough to make you scream. I suffered with my low-carb pancakes, looking enviously at the traditional ones the rest of my family was enjoying—until I discovered this recipe. Saturday mornings were beautiful once again!

Low-Carb Maple Pecan Pancakes[9]
Recipe by George Stella

Ingredients

    Nonstick cooking spray or butter

    2 eggs

    1/3 cup heavy cream

    1/4 cup water

    1 teaspoon no-sugar-added maple extract

    1/2 cup soy flour

    2 tablespoons sugar substitute (recommended: Splenda)

    1 tablespoon wheat (or oat) bran

    1/4 teaspoon baking powder

    1/8 cup chopped pecans (walnuts may be substituted)

Instructions

    Grease a griddle or large pan with nonstick cooking spray or butter and heat over medium heat. Mix all ingredients except pecans in a blender for about 15 seconds. Stop and scrape down the sides with a spatula, and continue mixing ingredients for another 15 seconds until well-blended.

    Pour approximately 16 mini-cakes onto the hot griddle

and sprinkle each with a few pecans. Cook on each side for only a minute or two. Serve hot with melted butter on top, or use a sugar-free syrup.

Cheesecake

There are a tremendous variety of low-carb cheesecakes available in books and on the Internet. This is my own favorite. It tastes so good you could forget it's treating your pancreas so gently.

Orange Sour-Cream Cheesecake with Chocolate Topping[10]

Crust ingredients

3/4 cup ground almonds (1-1/2 cups before grinding)

1 teaspoon grated orange peel

4 packets Splenda

3 tablespoons unsalted butter

Preheat oven to 350°F.

Mix Splenda and orange peel with ground almonds; set aside. Melt butter in microwave or on stovetop, then add to nut mixture and stir until evenly distributed. Spray 9-inch pie plate or small springform pan with cooking spray. Pat nut mixture into pie plate or pan, using a spoon or fingers, to cover bottom and sides. (During baking, it's a good idea to put a cookie sheet under a springform pan to stop butter from dripping on the bottom of your oven and making a mess.) Bake for 10 to 12 minutes, being careful not to overcook. Cool on a wire rack.

Filling ingredients

2 8-oz packages cream cheese

1/2 cup sour cream

3/4 cup Splenda

1-1/2 teaspoons pure orange extract (or 1/2 teaspoon orange oil)

2 eggs

Preheat oven to 350°F.

Combine cream cheese, sour cream, Splenda, and extract or oil in food processor until creamy and smooth. Add eggs and process until well-blended. Alternatively, mix with standard mixer. (If you use this method, cream cheese and eggs should be room temperature to avoid lumps.)

Pour into cooled crust and bake at 350°F for approximately 40 minutes or until center is mostly set (the center should still jiggle a little when you take it out of the oven). Bake times will vary depending on ovens and the type of pan used.

Allow to cool for 30 minutes on wire rack. Transfer to refrigerator and chill, covered, 6 to 8 hours or overnight.

Topping ingredients

1/2 cup sour cream

4 packets Splenda

1 teaspoon pure orange extract (or 2 drops orange oil)

1 low-carb or sugar-free dark chocolate bar

1/8 cup sliced almonds

In a small bowl, combine first three ingredients and whisk

until well blended. Spread on top of chilled cheesecake. Refrigerate for 1 to 2 hours, covered.

Just before removing the mixture from refrigerator, melt chocolate bar in microwave until it resembles a chocolate sauce, but try to avoid letting it bubble or boil. Cool for approximately 30 seconds. Remove cheesecake from refrigerator; drizzle top with chocolate to decorate. Quickly sprinkle with almonds while chocolate is still soft.

This stores refrigerated up to 10 days, or frozen for up to 3 months.

Serves 10 to 11 people with 7.6 net grams of carbohydrate per serving.

Low-Carb Muffins

Low-carb muffins are my frequent dinner companions. They take the place of rolls, at a fraction of the cost. No recipe here. Just buy the mixes you can find at your regular grocery store or health-food store. Follow the directions and enjoy!

Dreamfields Pasta

Another product I forced myself to live with in the early days was the absolutely yukky-tasting low-carb pastas. Sure they were low-carb, but did they have paid researchers working feverishly to make sure they tasted so miserable? Then I discovered Dreamfields brand pastas. These pastas are made with premium durum wheat semolina, but have been fashioned in such a way that fewer carbs get absorbed into your system. As a result they taste just like the real deal, but your blood sugars don't skyrocket. What a blessing. Spaghetti is back on the menu! For true diabetics, you need to test the effects of these pastas with your glucometer just to make sure your body doesn't overreact to them. But most of us can enjoy pasta again without guilt!

Natural Ovens Bakery Bagels

Bagels are one of the worst high-carb foods you can eat. Filled with lots of thick, doughy, white flour, they contain more carbs than most candy bars. Low-carb bagels exist, but they are harder to find than many other low-carb products. For a guy like me who travels, bagels are a great companion. They can handle a few bumps and bruises they might get in my carry-on luggage, and they are a great foundation for a spread of peanut butter or cream cheese.

Most of the low-carb bagels I've had tasted pretty good, but the Natural Ovens Bakery bagels taste awesome. Not only are they "as good" as regular; in my book they are considerably better. And they have only seven net carbs per bagel. Now the bad news. You can't find them in most stores. Check with your grocer. If you can't get them locally, you can order them at www.naturalovens.com. The shipping is expensive if you just order one package, so order several packages and freeze the ones you won't be using soon.

Bluebunny Ice-Cream Bars

These ice-cream bars are indistinguishable from the old-fashioned kind, but they have a skimpy four net carbs per bar (they're sweetened with Splenda). Add a handful of peanuts, fix a cup of gourmet coffee, put on a DVD of *Casablanca,* and you have a sweet night.

Homemade Ice-Cream Sundaes

You can't do better than this. This is my favoritest, bestest dessert of all![11]

"Dennis's Favorite" mock vanilla ice cream[12]

1 cup heavy cream

1/2 cup sugar substitute (recommended: Splenda)

1-1/2 teaspoons no-sugar-added vanilla extract

2 tablespoons whole-milk ricotta cheese

With an electric mixer on high, whip the heavy cream in a bowl just until frothy. Add in the sugar substitute, vanilla, and ricotta cheese, and continue to whip on high until peaks form. Be careful not to overwhip, or cream will break.

Using a 3-ounce ice-cream scoop, place a scoop in a champagne glass. Freeze to make faux ice cream, or serve refrigerated as a parfait.

Using this "ice cream" as your base, you can then add a few strawberries (don't buy the packages that have sugar added), break up about half of a low-carb chocolate bar, and mix in a few almonds. You'll have a "sundae" that is absolutely awesome. (One trick you can play—make this and serve it to guests who have been skeptical about low-carb eating. Don't tell them these are low-carb until after they have remarked about how fantastic they are!)

Low-Carb Strawberry-Cream Pie[13]

This is another one of those desserts that makes you

forget you're eating low-carb. One of my co-workers was eating with me at a church social. When he saw me eating this dessert, his curiosity got the best of him and he went back for a helping. After tasting it he said, "I used to feel sorry for Dennis with his low-carb eating, but not any more!"

Meringue shell

4 egg whites

1/4 teaspoon cream of tartar

3 tablespoons Splenda

Filling

1 small pkg. sugar-free gelatin (strawberry or raspberry)

1 pint heavy cream

1 8-oz. pkg. cream cheese, softened

1/4 cup Splenda

1 quart strawberries, cleaned and sliced

Preheat oven to 275°F. Grease one Pyrex pie plate and set aside. Beat egg whites until foamy. Add cream of tartar, then beat until whites stand in peaks. Add Splenda and beat for an additional minute or two.

Spread the meringue evenly in the bottom of the plate and up the sides.

Bake 1 hour and 10 minutes in a 275° F oven, then raise the temperature to 300° and bake for an additional 20 minutes. Remove from oven and cool while you make filling.

Dissolve gelatin with 3/4 cup boiling water. Stir in 1/3 cup cold water. Place in freezer for approximately 15 to

20 minutes (just until it begins to gel). When the gelatin is ready, whip the heavy cream until stiff (but not dry). Fold in cream cheese and Splenda. Fold in gelatin.

Stir in strawberries (reserving a few for garnish if desired). Pour over meringue shell in pie plate and let chill until firm—about 2 hours.

Five grams per serving.

Note: I like this pie better when the nutty shell below is substituted for the meringue shell given above.

Ingredients

2/3 cup soy flour

1/2 cup finely ground pecans

1/3 cup whole-grain pastry flour

1/4 cup Splenda

6 tablespoons chilled butter, cut into 12 pieces

2 tablespoons ice water

Directions

Heat oven to 425°F. In a large bowl combine together soy flour, pecans, pastry flour, and sugar substitute. Mix in butter with a pastry blender until butter pieces are about the size of peas. Add the ice water; stir to combine.

Transfer crust mixture to a 9-inch pie plate. Press along bottom and sides of pie plate to form a crust. Place in freezer to harden for around 15 minutes.

Cover crust with aluminum foil and bake 15 minutes; remove from oven and take off foil.

Finally, let me remind you that the Internet is bursting with all kinds of low-carb recipes. So are the bookstores. The knowledge you need to make your life a little easier and a lot nicer is there for you. Investigate. Enjoy. And thank God for the knowledge He has made available and the blessings of health.

Notes

1. Michael Eades, *Protein Power* (New York: Bantam Books, 1997), p. 22.
2. *New England Journal of Medicine,* March 28, 1991.
3. Eades, p. 172.
4. Eades, p. 323.
5. Eades, p. 24.
6. Dr. Joseph Mercola, www.mercola.com.
7. National Institute of Diabetes & Digestive & Kidney Diseases, "Diabetes Prevention Study Benefits American Indian Participants," www.niddk.nih.gov/welcome/releases/02-06-2002.htm.
8. Eades.
9. www.foodnetwork.com.
10. www.lowcarbluxury.com.
11. www.foodnetwork.com.
12. By George Stella. Check out George's excellent TV program, *Low Carb and Lovin' It,* on the Food Network.
13. www.recipegal.com.

About Spirit of Grace Ministries

Spirit of Grace Ministries is dedicated to spiritual renewal in the church and spiritual awakening in the world. Through conferences, evangelistic meetings, and the production of articles and books, the ministry is committed to promoting the principles and truths that lead to a greater awareness of the gospel of Jesus Christ and the presence and power of the Holy Spirit.

Dennis Pollock serves as the evangelist for Spirit of Grace Ministries. Since his early days as a Christian he has passionately studied topics such as revival, the role of the Holy Spirit in the life of the believer, Bible prophecy, prayer, and evangelism. After many years of intensive study of these issues and their practical application in ministry (which Dennis did as a pastor and then as an associate with Lamb & Lion Ministries), Dennis was called by God to teach these things to the body of Christ. God also called Dennis to preach in evangelistic missions all over the world, especially in Africa.

You can learn more about Spirit of Grace Ministries at their Web site: www.sogmin.org. If your church or organization would like to have Dennis come and teach on the subjects mentioned above (and perhaps add a talk on runaway blood sugar, the topic of this book), you can reach him by e-mail at dpollock@sogmin.org.

If you would like to be on Dennis's mailing list to receive his free monthly newsletter, just send an e-mail with your street address or PO box, or write to—

Spirit of Grace Ministries
PO Box 2068
McKinney TX 75070

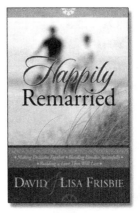

Happily Remarried

Making Decisions Together
Blending Families Successfully
Building a Love That Will Last
DAVID AND LISA FRISBIE

In North America today, nearly 60 percent of remarriages end in divorce. In *Happily Remarried*, you'll find ways to build the long-term unity that will keep your relationship from becoming just another statistic.

From more than 20 years of speaking, teaching, and counseling, David and Lisa Frisbie understand the situations you face every day. Using many examples drawn from real-life remarriages, they speak with hope and humor about the challenges, leading you through...

- *four key strategies:* forgiving everyone, having a "forever" mind-set, using conflict to get better acquainted, and forming a spiritual connection around God
- *practical marriage-saving advice* on where to live, discipline styles, kids and their feelings, "ex's," and finances
- *questions for discussion and thought* that will help you talk through and think over how the book's advice can apply to *your* circumstances

Combined with the indispensable ingredient of Scripture-based counsel, all of this makes for a great how-to recipe for a successful, happy remarriage.

~ Includes Helpful Discussion Guide ~

When Pleasing Others
Is Hurting You

Finding God's Patterns
for Healthy Relationships
DAVID HAWKINS

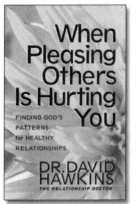

You want to do the right thing—take care of your family, be a good employee, "be there" for your friends. And you're good at it. Everyone knows they can depend on you—so they do.

But are you really doing what's best for them? And what about you? Are you growing? Are you happy and relaxed? Are you excited about your gifts and your calling, or do you sometimes think...*I don't even know what I want anymore.*

In this engaging and provocative book, psychologist David Hawkins will show you why you feel driven to always do more. You'll see how you can actually lose vital parts of your personality and shortchange God's work in your life. And you'll be inspired to rediscover the person God created you to be.

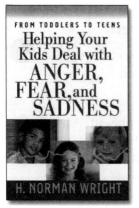

Helping Your Kids Deal with Anger, Fear, and Sadness

BY H. NORMAN WRIGHT

No parents wants to see their child struggle, especially with dark emotions such as anger, fear, and sadness. It's difficult to admit your child might be oppressed by these feelings, but this book can help. Family counselor and bestselling author Norm Wright addresses these emotional issues in a compassionate, family-friendly way that will enable you as a parent to bring comfort and a fresh perspective to your child.

Included in this interactive manual are conversational guidelines and learning activities for children that will encourage them to work through their difficult emotions. You as a parent will gain keen insights into the cause of these intense moods and be able to develop sound principles in dealing effectively with them.

Biblically-based and solution-oriented, *Helping Your Kids Deal with Anger, Fear, and Sadness* is an invaluable tool for parents who want to help their children and love and understand them better.

When Your Past Is Hurting Your Present

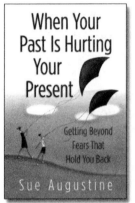

Getting Beyond Fears That Hold You Back

SUE AUGUSTINE

Is your past dictating your present? And your future? Do you want to break this destructive pattern and move on to a happier life, but find it impossible to do so?

Sue Augustine understands your situation. She too was once held captive by a painful past. With compassion, empathy, and a touch of humor, Sue shows you how to...

- identify, release, and change how you respond to the past
- overcome a "victim" stance
- trade bitterness and resentment for peace and joy
- set goals for the future with passion and purpose
- understand God's incredible timing and direction

If you're struggling with a difficult past that's harming your present and crippling your future, you can begin today to cut loose the baggage of the long-ago...and start to see your fears conquered, your dreams renewed, and your future become bright with new possibilities.